D1470387

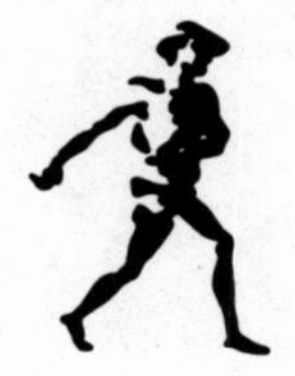

Other Books by Helen Neal:

Better Communications for Better Health (editor)
The Politics of Pain

What You Can Do to Preserve—and Even Enhance—Your Usable Sight

LOW VISION

by Helen Neal

Introduction by August Colenbrander, M.D.
Chairman, Committee on Low Vision,
American Academy of Ophthalmology

SIMON AND SCHUSTER
NEW YORK

Published by Simon and Schuster
A Division of Simon & Schuster, Inc.
Simon & Schuster Building
Rockefeller Center
1230 Avenue of the Americas
New York, New York 10020

Designed by Eve Kirch
Manufactured in the United States of America

3 5 7 9 10 8 6 4 2

Library of Congress Cataloging in Publication Data

Neal, Helen.
Low vision.

Bibliography: p.
Includes index.
1. Vision disorders. 2. Vision disorders—
Patients—Rehabilitation. 3. Vision disorders—
Patients—Services for. I. Title. [DNLM:
1. Vision Disorders. WW 140 N339L]
RE91.N4 1987 617.7 86-31406
ISBN: 0-671-52379-1

CONTENTS

ACKNOWLEDGMENTS

British journalist William Bolitho once said there are just two sorts of people: fountains and wells, givers and takers. It was my good fortune during the preparation of this book to encounter a preponderance of fountains, men and women who enthusiastically shared knowledge, ideas and opinions.

I first heard about low vision services in 1981, and at that time I realized that this was a new frontier in eye care. But few people, including many eye-care specialists, knew anything about low vision. There were only two books on the subject, both by and for clinicians. I began my quest with an inquiry to a local optometric association, which referred me to Dr. Michael J. Weitz, one of the few low vision specialists in the Washington, D.C., area. He in turn introduced me to Dr. Norman E. Wallis, executive director of the National Board of Examiners in Optometry—the first instance of good luck that marked my quest. Former president of the Pennsylvania College of Optometry, Dr. Wallis has been an early advocate of low vision services and was the moving spirit behind the founding of the college's Eye Institute, opened in 1978, with its keystone the William Feinbloom Vision Rehabilitation Center, now world-renowned for its low vision services. Dr. Wallis wholeheartedly endorsed my project for writing a book on low vision, referred me to leaders in the low vision field throughout the country, and in the ensuing months generously served as an adviser. I am deeply indebted to Dr. Wallis for setting my course and for his continuing help and encouragement.

I soon realized how little I knew about low vision and that there was a dearth of published information. My orientation began with "tutorial" sessions, interviews with "teachers" who gave me an overview of low vision services, putting them into historical and professional context. I am pleased to acknowledge here the contributions made to this book by Dr. William V. Padula, then national consultant on low vision for the American Foundation for the Blind; Marvin Brotman, founder and past president of the Council of Citizens with Low Vision; and Dr. Kenneth J. Myers, director of Optometric Service in the Veterans Administration's Department of Medicine and Surgery, an authority on vision rehabilitation services pioneered by the Veterans Administration following World War II. With the thorough background provided by these tutors, I was able to organize my research. I hope the publication of this book will make them feel their time with me was well spent.

I am especially grateful to the directors and members of their staffs in the low vision clinics I visited in the United States, Canada and England. Information I obtained during these visits is distilled in Chapter Four of this book, which I consider the heart of the book. The extraordinary cooperation of these practitioners—doctors, instructors in the use of low vision aids, social workers and patient advocates—was partly motivated by their conviction that the time had come for a book on low vision, one that would explain the new speciality to the general public, including the millions of partially sighted who would benefit from these services if they knew about them. To this end these professionals interrupted busy schedules and generously spent countless hours with me. My sense of obligation to them is limitless.

Throughout the years in which this book was in preparation, my chief mentor was James G. Chandler, former university librarian who, after retirement, crusaded for "access to information" by the visually impaired. To this end he developed voice-indexing techniques for recorded materials and promoted the use of high technology by the blind and those with partial sight. He was a major sounding board for me, and on many occasions his wise counsel kept me from being victimized by my enthusiasms. Over the years, this "fountain" kept me informed of developments on all fronts, the politics of blindness, changes in programs for the partially sighted, trends and training. To this wise and generous man I gratefully acknowledge my indebtedness.

Members of the National Eye Institute staff were a vital source of information on current vision research, especially Dr. Constance W. Atwell, who provided ready answers to my numerous questions and brought to my attention significant research studies and reports of meetings. And to Joel Sugarman, information specialist with the Eye Institute, I am most grateful for his patience and efficiency over the years in responding to my many requests for statistics and other information.

Among former colleagues at the National Institutes of Health who were part of an informal news network, I single out for special thanks Marc A. Stern, chief of the News Branch of the Public Information Service, not only for his providing me with vision-related information, but for his unfailing interest in the book and for his encouragement.

Fortunate is the author blessed with a good editor. Bob Bender, senior editor at Simon and Schuster, is living proof that there are some ideal editors left in the publishing business. Over the years, we made our way by phone through the manuscript, chapter by chapter, in accordance with his editorial system, as I mailed him each chapter when I finished it. After he had edited and returned the chapter, over the phone we discussed his changes and suggestions, a system that precluded major surprises about content in the finished manuscript. The only negative aspect to this long-distance system was that it deprived me of an editor-author lunch in a fancy New York restaurant. It was a pleasure working with such a top-flight editor, who believed in the importance of the book and was always accessible and understanding. I am most grateful to him not only for his editorial expertise, but for his courteous guidance from book proposal to publication.

Dr. Joanne Economon, an ophthalmologist who combines eye surgery with low vision services in her practice, from the beginning provided an attentive ear and sound professional advice. And to my good friend and kindred spirit, author Melanie Choukas-Bradley, I am indebted for helping me surmount bouts of writer frustration, blocks, and those periods when the brain sags and the computer breaks down.

It is a pleasure to acknowledge the help given me by Patricia M. Beattie, community consultant with the Mid-Atlantic Region of the American Foundation for the Blind, and Laura Oftedahl, director of public affairs for the American Council for the Blind. Throughout the preparation of the book these two women provided a flow of reference materials. I am especially grateful to Laura for her help in the preparation of the resources section of the book.

Among those who were part of my informal information network, I single out Vivian Dickson and Wanda Warddell, former colleagues at the National Institutes of Health, who alerted me to pertinent articles in professional journals. And my special thanks to Gail Reardon for her diligence, days, nights and weekends, typing final drafts of chapters as I came down to each chapter deadline.

To the numerous "fountains"—practitioners, scientists, administrators, manufacturers of products for the partially sighted, numerous partially sighted men and women who shared their experiences with me, and to good friends—who in many ways contributed so generously to this book, I give my heartfelt collective thanks.

To
My Dear Friend and Niece
Patricia Neal Emsellem

INTRODUCTION

by August Colenbrander, M.D., Chairman, Committee on Low Vision, American Academy of Ophthalmology

How concerned should one be about a scar $\frac{1}{16}$ of an inch in length? On most areas of our body the result would be hardly noticeable. But if this scar is located in the macula, the center of the back of the eye, the result can be devastating. This example demonstrates the extraordinary importance of our eyes relative to the rest of our body. For most of our daily activities vision is of vital importance. Our eyes, one inch in diameter, send more information to our brain than all other senses combined, and most of that information is processed through a small central area responsible for our sharpest detail vision. Even the IRS recognizes the special role of vision and grants a tax deduction for "legal blindness," a deduction not available for any other loss of bodily function. No wonder that for many people the loss of sight seems as fearsome as the loss of life itself.

At one time it was useful to characterize the health of a population by its death rate. Today, we have become more interested in the quality of life of those living. Once it was appropriate to characterize the level of eye care by counting those who are "blind." Today, we recognize that it is not only the blind who ask for our attention; equally important is the much larger group in the gray area between normal vision and blindness. This gray area is appropriately described by the words *low vision*—"low" because there is less than normal vision, and "vision" because we are definitely not dealing with blindness.

To gain a better understanding of vision loss and its many aspects it is helpful to consider the key words *disorder, impairment, disability* and *handicap.* These words are not just interchangeable synonyms. *Disorder* describes a change in the orderly anatomical structure, in our example a scar on the macula. *Impairment* measures the resulting functional deficit, in our example a loss of the ability to see detail (visual acuity) and a gap (blind spot) in the central area of the visual field. Such measures describe how the eye functions, but they do not necessarily indicate how the individual can function. An individual with loss of one eye, for instance, can function almost normally in most regards. *Dis-ability* describes the effect on the abilities of the individual. In our example the individual would be unable to read a distant road sign or to read newsprint without a magnifier. *Handicap,* finally, describes how this lack of abilities affects the person's position in society.

Low vision is not a single condition, just as sickness is not a single disease. To alleviate their burden, patients with low vision need care in many different areas. Underlying disorders need to be treated. This is the domain of medical and surgical care provided by ophthalmologists. Impairments can often be reduced with glasses and other optical aids. This is the domain of ophthalmologists and optometrists. Abilities must be enhanced through education and training. This is the domain of teachers of the visually handicapped, including orientation and mobility instructors. Finally, the patients' handicap must be reduced by providing a setting for vocational and daily living activities in which their abilities are optimized while their disabilities are minimized. This is the domain of vocational counselors and placement services. No one professional could provide this full spectrum of services. Low vision requires a broad range of expertise from various professionals. While multidisciplinary teamwork is not always easy to achieve, this book gives vivid testimony that many individuals in a variety of settings are striving toward this goal. The goal is still far from being reached, but we need to acknowledge the enormous shift in awareness that has occurred in the last quarter-century as we set out for the next. This book will undoubtedly raise the awareness of all concerned: of patients and their relatives; of educators and employers; and last but not least, of the health-care professionals.

1

The "Discovery" of Low Vision

Now that life expectancy in the United States has climbed to seventy-five years, American eyes, forced to work longer, are not up to it. At the turn of the century, when the average life span of Americans was forty-seven years, eyesight, as if designed by nature for a photofinish, usually lasted a lifetime. But in this era of sight-demanding technology and high speed, when reading and viewing occupies so much of our business and leisure time, and when aging takes its visual toll, American eyes, forced to work almost thirty years longer than those of their forebears, can't cope with the added demands.

Half the population wears eyeglasses or contact lenses. American consumers spend about $6.6 billion annually for conventional eyewear. Those whose vision is improved by this type of eyewear are the lucky ones.

An estimated 11.4 million Americans have impaired vision that cannot be improved by conventional eyeglasses or contact lenses. These are the "hard of seeing," most of them elderly, who resign themselves to squinting at television and at labels in the supermarket, who write illegible letters to their children and friends, can't see traffic lights distinctly, and have given up reading. Visually impaired teenagers quit school and take menial jobs that do not require good vision. Nursing homes are filled with older men and women who couldn't cope with living in a world they saw only as a blur. Many parents of children born with cataracts and other visual defects reluctantly put those children into schools for the blind without knowing how much usable vision they have or what surgery and other medical treatment could do to correct the defects.

In the business world, to admit that one's vision is failing can result in being fired or transferred to a lower-paying job in which one's skills and experience are wasted. Young and old resort to all sorts of ruses to conceal their severe visual defects. A young assistant director in a large public agency, who could not admit even to herself that her vision was failing, pretended in staff meetings to read reports passed out for comment. Back in her office, she would ask a co-worker to read the reports to her, explaining her inability to read it with "I lost one of my contact lenses" or "I have a slight eye infection" or "I broke my glasses on my way to the office." In classrooms, some partially sighted children, rather than admit openly that they can't see the writing on the blackboard, prefer to be labeled stupid.

No one knows the number of "visual closet cases" or even how many partially sighted people there are in the United States. But estimates of those with severe eye defects ranging from partial sight to total blindness have been put as high as 11.4 million, including the 500,000 certified as legally blind by eye doctors.

The medical definition of blindness is the inability to perceive light. How many totally blind are there in the United States? The estimate is 50,000 of the 500,000 certified as legally blind. The remaining 450,000 have some residual vision, 85 percent with usable vision. The term "legal blindness" started out as "economic blindness" during the Great Depression, when federal projects put millions of unemployed to work on public-works projects. On the edges of this massive emergency job operation were the blind. Traditionally cared for by private charities, churches or their own families, or supporting themselves by begging on the streets, the blind found themselves in economic limbo.

At the request of the federal government, the American Medical Association came up with a definition of "economic blindness"—that is, visual impairment that prevented men and women from seeing well enough to work. The Social Security Board changed that term to "legal blindness" and set numerical visual measurements as a basis of eligibility for financial and other benefits.

Only recently have those arbitrary standards come

under fire. Unchanged in half a century, they are still used by government and private agencies to define "legal blindness." Ophthalmologist Dr. Eleanor E. Faye says in her book *Clinical Low Vision:*

> *Legal blindness* is an outmoded term that, in most states in the United States and in some other countries, incorporates the assumption that on the basis of a corrected visual acuity of 20/200 or less and a field of 20 degrees or less, *without any functional evaluation,* a person can be classified as legally blind. When a person meets these arbitrary standards, he becomes eligible for an extra income-tax deduction and he can get job training and special education benefits from the state, but he also can receive a "blindness" label that automatically segregates him from sighted people on a technicality rather than on the basis of a functional assessment; his infirmity becomes a matter of public record. Many working people do not want to be classified as legally blind for fear that their employers will find out and fire them on this technicality rather than keep them because of the quality of their work.

Dr. Samuel M. Genensky, like Dr. Faye, an active leader in the low vision services movement and director of the Center for the Partially Sighted in Santa Monica, California, says:

> The vast majority of the legally blind are not blind. They are able, with the help of appropriate visual aids, to use their remaining eyesight to read ordinary ink-printed material, write with pen or pencil, and move about with-

out the help of a cane, guide dog, or sighted companion. Most partially sighted persons, whether legally blind or not, will never become functionally blind.

We have tended to offer the partially sighted either no services at all or services developed for the totally blind. We have said, "Go away. You have too much sight to deserve help." Or, "We will help you only if you will totally disregard or completely discount your remaining eyesight." Only recently have we begun to recognize the partially sighted as an entity distinct from the blind and to provide services for them.

Low vision as a special category received official recognition in the Ninth Edition of the International Classification of Diseases published every ten years by the World Health Organization. In previous editions only blindness was codified. "One was either blind or sighted," says Dr. August Colenbrander, medical director of Low Vision Services at the Pacific Medical Center in San Francisco and member of the committee that prepared the Ninth Edition, published in 1979.

> There was no recognition of the wide range of degrees of sightedness we know now from low vision testing methods. My collaborators and I were able to convince the editors that low vision is a special category that should be identified as such. As a result, for the first time low vision is codified in the International Classification of Diseases.

"Low vision" as defined by the National Eye Institute—and in this book—means that a person, even with the help of corrective glasses or contact lenses, cannot read newspaper type or a sign on a bus or labels on canned goods, or recognize friends in the street. The major causes of low vision in adults are macular degeneration, glaucoma, diabetic retinopathy and cataracts. Some children are born with cataracts and glaucoma, but common causes of low vision in children are *amblyopia* ("lazy eye"), *strabismus* (crossed eyes), *myopia,* and *retinopathy of prematurity,* a retinal disorder of premature infants. What can be done to enhance the vision of the millions whose severe visual defects cannot be corrected by conventional eyewear? What new methods of visual assessment, diagnosis and treatment can be applied to them?

In the late 1950s these questions were addressed by a few eye specialists, scientists, surgeons and optical experts, as well as Veterans Administration doctors who were dealing with thousands of veterans blinded in the Second World War. About that time, a new concept of vision was developed, a revolutionary idea that shifted emphasis from blindness to sightedness by advocating the maximum use of whatever vision a person had. Advocates of this new concept—which today we recognize as the low vision movement— were optometrists and ophthalmologists who, in their daily practice, using new diagnostic and vision assessment techniques, were discovering that many of their patients certified as legally blind actually had varying degrees of usable sight.

They found that standard visual-acuity tests of a person's ability to read letters of varying sizes at specified distances failed to assess a person's functional vision, the visual capacity to see in all weathers, to perform in kitchens or in classrooms, in an office or in a supermarket, to see a television screen, or to recognize friends (or enemies) at cocktail parties. The standard visual-acuity tests did not assess how well patients performed in everyday situations. How much of your day do you spend sitting bolt upright in a chair anchored to the floor, staring at rows of letters on a lighted chart?

The concept of using residual vision to the maximum surfaced in the United States at a time when severe visual defects were escalating. Of the many reasons for this escalation, chiefly was the growth of the population—more people, more eyes, more problems. The country had become a nation of survivors, beneficiaries of superb public-health systems, health education, and biomedical research that improved surgical and medical treatment of the eyes. Americans living well into their seventh and eighth decades often pay a price for those added years—chronic diseases and impaired eyesight. At the other end of the age scale, babies who might otherwise have died shortly after birth, were being saved by surgery and new methods of infant care. But the dark side of these life-saving measures is the number of children surviving with multiple disabilities, including defective sight. An increase in the number of head injuries caused by car crashes and other accidents and by street violence added to the case loads of hospital ophthalmologic departments.

Perhaps because it's a new category, low vision is variously, but seldom precisely, defined. But the essence of what eye specialists say about it is that those who have severely impaired but usable vision can enhance it with special optical and nonoptical aids, by modifying the home and work environment, and by mobility training. Low vision services are aimed at helping the partially sighted use to best advantage whatever vision they have.

Aging and the Partially Sighted

The 1960s saw an explosion of interest in vision. There were new organizations—most notably the National Eye Institute, established by Congress in 1968 as part of the National Institutes of Health. There were new diagnostic tools—at Johns Hopkins Medical School, Dr. Louise Sloan, a scientist specializing in visual psychophysics, was taking a critical look at traditional methods of measuring vision. Finding those methods inadequate for assessing functional vision, she developed distance-acuity charts and reading-text cards, designed optical aids, and set up a low vision clinic, one of the first in the country.

In this same decade, manufacturing companies were discovering the market for eye-care products—diagnostic instruments, pharmaceuticals and optical aids. High-tech industries entered the field with electronic equipment, special cameras connected to video screens that enabled the partially sighted to read ordinary-size type by magnifying it on the screen as much as sixty times its original size.

In the vanguard of the low vision movement, a cadre of optometrists and ophthalmologists quietly and without fanfare, set up clinics. As word spread, mostly by patients, they were inundated with requests for services. Through the services themselves, these eye-care specialists were changing the lives of people—many of whom had thought they were blind—by using new techniques for the assessment of remaining vision and prescribing aids custom-tailored to the visual need of each patient. Going beyond traditional eye examinations, these low vision specialists encompassed "the person behind the eyeballs," the whole person plagued by an array of social and psychological problems related to their defective vision.

In low vision clinics, doctors and therapists listened to what patients said about their reasons for wanting to improve their vision, their incentives to be self-reliant, earn a living, or catch the right bus to take them to work or downtown to shop. They also heard with considerable professional embarrassment accounts of patients being dismissed by other eye doctors with "There's nothing more that can be done for you. You'll just have to live with poor vision."

That attitude is not prevalent among low vision specialists. Their concern is not limited to their individual patients; it goes beyond to the millions of Americans who are not *blind,* but just can't see well with conventional lenses. "Historically," says Dr. Gerald R. Friedman, director of Low Vision Services at the Eye Research Institute of Retina Foundation in Boston,

> these people would have been considered to have inadequate vision for functioning in the sighted world and would have been classified as blind. Today we are in the fortunate position of being able to offer them a much better future. First, we call their condition "low vision," not blindness, and second—of far greater importance—we can offer low vision people the means of utilizing whatever vision they have left, no matter how great or how little that may be. In a visually oriented society, this can be the difference between independence and dependence, of being a productive part of society, not a victim of it.

Here was a new way of looking at the eyes, shifting the perspective from defects to prospects, a means of salvaging careers, talent and experience. Children who a decade or so before would have been shunted into schools for the blind could attend school with sighted classmates and, using special visual aids and training, keep up with them. Thousands of older men and women, handicapped in a bustling sighted world by their defective vision and unaware that it could be improved by low vision services, were reluctantly entering nursing homes, exchanging personal freedom for costly, debilitating custodial care.

Today the American Academy of Ophthalmology and the American Optometric Association have special sections on low vision. All colleges of optometry train their students in low vision services, and many have low vision clinics associated with their schools. In 1983 the Pennsylvania College of Optometry inaugurated this country's first graduate course in vision rehabilitation to prepare professionals from many disciplines for careers in or related to low vision. The announcement of the course brought inquiries from all over the United States and several foreign countries. In 1984, the first Master of Science degrees in vision rehabilitation were awarded in this pioneering graduate training program.

Despite obstacles, open and covert resistance from eye-care practitioners and agencies for the blind, low vision services have been putting down strong, deep roots. By 1986 there were hundreds of low vision clinics in schools of optometry, hospitals and eye institutes, and as free-standing units. Characteristic of any evolving specialty, diversity abounds in type of facility, methods of diagnosis and treatment, and in the composition of professional and back-up staffs. Clinics I visited in the United States, Canada and Great Britain ranged from a service run by an optical-aid technician in cramped quarters grudgingly allotted by a major eye institute not much interested in low vision, to a clinic occupying attractive, spacious, specially designed quarters with a multidisciplinary team of optometrists and ophthalmologists, therapists, trainers in the use of aids and in mobility and daily living skills, psychologists, and counselors for patients and their families. Large or small, these clinics are booked weeks, sometimes months in advance.

Unfortunately, few health- and medical-insurance policies pay for low vision assessments or for visual aids and training in their use. Neither does Medicare. Consequently, clients of low vision clinics are largely from middle and upper economic ranks who can pay for the services and special aids. While honoring the long-standing medical tradition of providing some free service to the indigent, most low vision clinics finance their operations with patients' fees and most have no difficulty balancing their budgets. But every clinic director I talked with deplored the lack of insurance payments for low vision services. As one director said, "The government hasn't caught up with the benefits of low vision services and what they are doing to keep thousands of men and women out of the blindness system. The hardest hit are older people living on small incomes, and they're the ones most afflicted by visual disorders that could be ameliorated."

As two million Americans turn sixty-five every year and 2,600,000 are in their eighties, the need for low vision services escalates. It's in the older age group that two thirds of serious visual problems occur. Though the government hasn't caught up with the facts, industry is well aware of them and is investing millions of dollars in the development of diagnostic and treatment equipment, optical and electronic aids, lens implants, and eye-care products. Says Henry Wendt, president of SmithKline, "There's no question about it, we're just beginning to discover the unlimited growth potential of the eye care industry." SmithKline is just one company that has invested heavily in the development of eye-care instrumentation.

Men and women crossing that sixty-five-year dateline these days don't conform to the stereotype of "old folks." Now it's Whistler's mother in designer jeans and Grandpa in his Dior jogging suit. These "young old" are not about to accept the label of blindness when their usable vision can be enhanced by special optical and nonoptical aids that enable them to keep good jobs or shift to new careers, trek around the world, return to school for degrees they missed out on, or find fulfillment in myriad other ways, expecting as confidently as they did in their youth that good things in life are coming to them.

What is sad is that so few of the visually impaired know about resources now available to them through low vision services. The clinics themselves, inundated by requests for their services, have tended to keep a low profile. I sensed in a few directors a desire not to antagonize eye-care professionals who regard low vision services as competition. But as Dr. Charles F. Mullen, executive director of the Philadelphia College of Optometry's Eye Institute said to me, "We believe in educating the public about the resources available to them. How can you help people if they don't know you exist?"

To make low vision services better known and to explain how this new specialty helps visually impaired children and adults is the purpose of this book.

2

How Do We See?

You've been looking at your face in mirrors for years —can you draw its likeness from memory? No matter that you can't draw a straight line (there are no straight lines in your face), can you see an image of your face in your mind's eye as if in a photograph? Visualizing your face, can you define its shape, whether it's round, square, oval or triangular? Your eyes—are they exactly the same size and shape? Which is the dominant eye? Is your nose aquiline, snub, broad, thin? Is your mouth thin and straight or full and sensuous? Does your chin jut or recede or form a gentle angle with your jaws? This exercise of visualizing your face from memory—first its separate parts then as the harmonious unit the world recognizes as *you*—may convince you that it's possible to "see" an object a thousand times without actually "seeing" it. This inability is no fault of your eyes, which may be in perfect working order, but it indicates that something other than the eyes themselves is involved in the seeing process.

Comparing your mental image of your face with a recent studio photograph, you most likely will discover some discrepancies between the two that account for your secret dislike of the photograph even though friends tell you it's a marvelous likeness. All of us have a mental image of our face, fixed in some period of our lives, usually in our youth, when we were more attractive than we may ever be again. Though outwardly we show signs of aging, that inner image remains relatively unchanged. Now and then we get a shock from an unexpected glimpse of our faces that we stubbornly refuse to acknowledge as a likeness.

The model used in describing how we see is most frequently the camera. There are similarities, to be sure, but that's because camera designers copied certain of nature's optical principles. In cameras and in the eyes, light is the activating element. Light enters the aperture of the camera and registers an image on film, and unless it's one of those "instant" cameras, its job is done. But the human eye goes far beyond registering an image on the "film" in its dark interior. Light, after passing through the cornea, pupil, lens, and the vitreous (the jellylike substance that keeps parts of the eye in place) hits the retina (that film scarlet with blood vessels) and is transformed into electrochemical signals that travel along strands in the optic nerve into the brain, the workshop where the business of seeing takes place.

Seeing is a learned activity. A baby does not see the minute it opens its eyes on the world. As every parent knows, the baby must learn to associate faces with the words *Mama* and *Daddy*. "We forget," says Dr. Joanne Economon, a Washington ophthalmologist specializing in low vision services,

> how hard it was for us as babies to learn to see. Adults blind since birth whose eye defects are corrected by surgery appreciate what babies go through learning to see. Adults who regain sight must also learn to see and they have just as hard a time of it. Even worse to some degree, because they must unlearn many of their sensory impressions of objects and the people around them.

Newly sighted adults, encountering the visual world for the first time, see a confusion of images and have difficulty deciding which objects to focus on, whether a door is more important than a wall, for instance. Even young adults who are born with sight, after losing it and not seeing for years, must get reacquainted with the visual world when sight is restored.

After the crash and explosion of his plane in the Korean War, Donald Garner, who later became director of Blind Rehabilitation Services of the Veterans Administration, was blind for seventeen years until, as a patient at the eye clinic of the National Institutes of Health, he underwent a series of operations that restored partial sight to one eye.

> I had to learn to adapt to a different visual environment after seventeen years of total blindness [he told me]. In those intervening years so much had changed, not only in cities that had once been familiar places, but in the pace of life itself. And other things, too. As I was flying home from the National Institutes of Health after the last operation that had restored partial sight, a flight attendant on the plane brought me some magazines. I was euphoric at the prospect of sitting there and reading like most of the other passengers. While I was blind I had listened to tapes of very interesting articles in *Playboy* magazine and when the attendant offered a stack of magazines, I selected *Playboy.* At last I'd be able to read articles I had only been able to listen to. You understand, I had never seen this magazine. I'll never forget my shock and embarrassment when, as I flipped it open, I saw the centerfold—a color photograph of a stark naked woman! And there was a flight attendant standing next to me. Yes, indeed, during those seventeen years I was blind, a lot had changed and not just the landscape.

When I was an art student studying portrait painting in New York, what fascinated me most was that, though every student was painting the same model, no two portraits resembled each other. In subsequent classes I discovered perceptual patterns among the students. There were students who distorted the model's features and those who idealized them. Instructors warned against these idiosyncrasies. "Don't make her so beautiful. She's just an ordinary-looking woman." One student who covered his canvas with the sweeping, broad brush strokes of a house painter was brought down with "It's not the broad brush, Albert. It's the broad mind!" And in every class there was that eerie phenomenon, the student who put on a distracting show of measuring the model's features, brush extended, one eye shut, and ended up with a self-portrait. What our instructors were trying to teach us was not so much how to put paint on canvas, but how to see beyond the limits of the eye, to see with our minds.

Others besides artists see with equal, if not artistic, intensity—city bus drivers for instance. Watch their eyes in the rear-view mirror, the ceaseless movement as the eyes assess traffic ahead, behind, and to the sides, judging a "stale" green traffic light two blocks ahead, spotting a car suddenly pulling away from the curb. Each second is a test of the driver's eye/brain visual system: a real test, not an eye examination in the quiet of an eye doctor's office, where the only task is to concentrate on reading without distraction the black letters on a lighted chart. What relation does such an eye examination have to the realities of driving a bus in rush-hour traffic? Very little. How many of us have the visual efficiency of bus drivers? The answer, of course, is in our dented fenders.

Sophisticated and brutal criminals will continue to be caught initially not by high-technology devices, such as instant computer retrieval of records and fingerprints or electronic listening, but by "the trained, discriminating human eye," says David Powis, deputy assistant commissioner of the London Metropolitan Police in his book *The Signs of Crime,* a manual for police officers. "Vigilance, or watchfulness, is a primary police quality, without which the other essential elements of the police officer's mental apparatus cannot function properly. Knowing what to watch for, however, is something that has to be learned." The ability to spot criminals on the street, Powis says, is an acquirable skill and "not innate detective ability or mysteriously recurring luck." This skill in spotting criminals on the street, in parking lots, and in buildings is one that private citizens are acquiring for survival in this era of ubiquitous crime.

An important element of seeing is the act of perceiving. Aldous Huxley in his book *The Art of Seeing* says that in the orthodox treatment of defective vision emphasis is placed on "only one element in the total process of seeing, namely the physiological mechanism of the sensing apparatus. Perception and the capacity to remember, upon which perception depends, are completely ignored." Considering the part the mind plays in the total visual process, treatment of defective vision, Huxley says, "must take account, not only of sensing but also of the process of remembering, without which perceiving is impossible."

Strong influences on how we perceive our personal world and the people in it are our prejudices and experience. An example of these influences on our perceptions is David Powis's comparison of the way police and victims perceive criminals and the perception of social workers, probation officers and lawyers who see criminals after they are caught,

> when they are defused and harmless. They hear their explanations when they [the criminals] are contrite, in sober clothes, accompanied by distraught relatives. Policemen, like victims of crime, see these greedy and sometimes violent thieves in a very different state. We see them when they are ruthless and aggressive or confidently arrogant; when they are fat and comfortable on the fruits of crime, telling us in obscene phrases to "prove it if you can."

Some people born with "super" vision come to our attention when success in their careers reveals their extraordinary eyesight. One such is Ted Williams, for many years a baseball star with the Boston Red Sox. His keen eyesight was legendary even before he retired. He used to boast that he could see the ball as it hit the bat. Teammates and others scoffed. As Ron Luciano recounts in *The Umpire Strikes Back,* Williams, challenged to prove his boast, in a demonstration on the practice field covered the barrel of his bat with tar and stepped up to the plate. When the first ball was pitched to him, he called out: "One seam!" as he hit. When the ball was retrieved, one seam was marked with tar. As one ball after another sped toward Williams at about ninety miles an hour and his bat struck them, he predicted the place on the ball that would reveal tar marks. "He called five out of seven perfectly," writes Luciano, "the most amazing display of hitting ability I've ever seen." At that time Williams was fifty-four years old.

Commercial photographers are generally among

those with exceptional visual acuity. But one sports photographer considered his 20/20 vision inadequate for his work. Distressed because he could no longer see the details of the string in basketball nets and fearing that his vision was declining, he went to a low vision clinic for an assessment. Tests showed he was right—his previous visual acuity of 20/15 had declined to 20/20. The low vision specialist prescribed an optical aid that brought his acuity up to 20/15.

Through the centuries learned men have theorized about the mechanics of seeing. Before the invention of the ophthalmoscope by Hermann Ludwig von Helmholtz in 1851 made possible the examination of the dark interior of the eyes (the pupil, which seems to be a flat black disk, is actually a "window"), scientists could only conjecture about the placement and functions of parts of the inner eye. Five hundred years ago, Leonardo da Vinci, in his remarkable treatise on optics, gave a clue to how the visual system works. Images, he wrote, pass through the center of the crystalline sphere situated in the middle of the eye (He was wrong about that, but who would quibble about such a mistake by that towering genius?) and in this center they unite in a point and then spread themselves out upon the opposite surface of this sphere and from thence they are transmitted to "the common sense where they are judged." The "common sense," he explained, is that which "judges the things given to it by the senses."

From da Vinci's research to exquisitely refined studies of the brain cells of the visual system was a five-hundred-year journey into the technology of modern science. In 1983, Drs. David H. Hubel and Torsten N. Wiesel received the Nobel Prize for their research, conducted twenty years before, on the visual system of the brain. In science, prestigious awards are never hasty things; there must be time for other scientists to prove new theories. But by the time Hubel and Wiesel received their award, some of their precepts were already being applied in correcting eye defects.

An incalculable benefit to children born blind from cataracts or blinded by injuries in infancy was the discovery by the two Nobelists that surgery should be performed as early as possible to correct the defects. The idea of operating on the eyes of a two-week-old baby would have seemed preposterous twenty years ago, but developments in anesthesiology and surgery make such operations feasible, and the findings of Hubel and Wiesel have made them imperative. The two scientists had discovered that unless cells in the baby's brain's visual system are properly stimulated by signals from the eyes, certain of those cells may "turn off" forever, impeding normal visual development. It had been commonplace medical practice to wait until children entered school before corrective eye surgery was performed. Drs. Hubel and Wiesel showed that such a delay was much too long and that an infant's brain, deprived of visual stimulation, would never catch up, never close the gap, and certain brain cells not nourished by visual images could atrophy.

A corollary to the findings of Drs. Hubel and Wiesel is the importance of exercising vision as early in life as possible. There is a lot to be said for all those mobiles flying over cribs and the little blue elephants chasing red butterflies over the wallpaper.

Do we need two eyes? It helps to have two working eyes. Beams of light entering each eye produce slightly different images in the brain's visual system where these images combine to give us accurate depth perception. But we can get along quite well with only one good eye, as Robert Wernick, who lost the sight of one eye from retinal detachment, explains in his article on "one-eyed jacks," published in *Smithsonian Magazine.* "A lifetime of experience is just as good as stereoscopic vision at telling me where objects are in space," Wernick says. With one eye, he can drive a car and hit a golf ball, but "children, bicycles, dogs did develop a way of turning up with disconcerting suddenness on my right, or blind side." Among famous "one-eyed jacks" is Lord Nelson, British naval hero, who, during an engagement with Danish ships, was ordered by his superior officer on a nearby ship to withdraw from battle. Nelson put his spyglass to his blind eye, saw no signal for withdrawal and went on to defeat the Danish fleet. In more recent times, the list of men who found their one-eyed status no hindrance to their careers includes Moshe Dayan, Sammy Davis, Jr., and Rex Harrison.

Those of us with two working eyes have a dominant eye. Can you tell by looking into a mirror which of your eyes is dominant? It's not easy to tell unless one eye is noticeably occluded by a drooping eyelid or is smaller than the other. Nor can we see both our eyes or those of anybody else simultaneously. We must shift our focus from one to the other to try to find the dominant eye. Most of us learn early on to fix our gaze on one eye when talking to people. Constantly shifting from one eye to another is disconcerting to the person we're looking at and, in our culture, shifty eyes supposedly denote a shifty character.

Portrait painters through the ages have intuitively selected the dominant eye for emphasis. Robert Henri, American painter and renowned teacher, called the attention of his students to the "compositional relation between the eyes—that is, one eye commands the greater interest. If you paint them equal, no matter what the position of the head, the observer will get no right conception of them. In life, one eye always dominates the observer. In painting this domination must persist."

There's more to the dominant eye than aesthetics. Physiologically the dominant eye is the "worker eye," the one we use unconsciously to do most of our seeing. Even some eye doctors have difficulty in determining which is the dominant eye. Dr. Joanne Economon uses a little ruse to test her patients. Without telling them what she's up to, she makes a pinhole in a three-by-five card, hands it to the patient and says: "Look through the pin hole." Invariably the patient puts the card up to the dominant worker eye.

Knowing which is the dominant eye has significance in eye surgery. In his book, *Cataracts: The Complete Guide—From Diagnosis to Recovery—For Patients and Families,* Dr. Julius Shulman says: "If a cataract develops in only one eye and that is your nondominant eye, you may not even know it is there until the vision in that eye is surprisingly poor. . . . If a choice were possible, it would be better to have a cataract in your nondominant eye." Unfortunately, we can't make that choice, but knowing which is the dominant eye can help us make decisions about the timing of cataract surgery.

Dr. Shulman suggests this test for finding your dominant eye:

> Bring together the tip of your thumb and forefinger into an "O," about six inches from your face. . . . Focus on an object across the room so that it is in the middle of the "O." Closing one eye and then the other will tell you which eye is dominant. If you close your left eye and the object is still in the center of the "O," then your right eye was the "sighting" eye and is the dominant one and vice versa.

In the course of mapping the brain's visual system, Drs. Hubel and Wiesel found that, when testing one eye and then the other with identical stimuli, the responses were different. In most instances, cells in one eye consistently produce a higher frequency of "firing" than in the other. Their studies revealed that, throughout the entire binocular part of the brain's visual fields, are neurons with all degrees of "eye preference," that is, preferring one eye to the other, a preference, the scientists postulated, that is encoded in the genes. Only when one eye monopolizes the eye work to an excessive degree can there be serious consequences. The non-dominant eye gives up trying to see. The result is a "lazy eye," or amblyopia, a defect that, if not corrected in early childhood, can result later on in blindness in that eye.

Can eye exercises improve vision? When I asked ophthalmologists and optometrists this question several recoiled, almost as if there were some indecency in the question. When pressed to explain their attitude, some admitted that there was a "crackpot" element in eye-exercise therapy that goes back several decades to extravagant claims by some therapists for systems that had little or no scientific basis.

At that time there were "seeing schools" in the United States, England and Germany that specialized in "reeducating the eyes." There are no data on how successful those schools were, but they faded away as research revealed new information about the physiology of the eyes themselves and their role as "outposts of the brain," not mindless surveillance cameras, but an integral, inseparable part of the eye/brain system. New technologies were coming up with instruments for assessing vision and the health of eyes. Attention was being focused on eye impairments in children and ways of measuring their visual acuity even before they could read letters. "Seeing schools" became obsolete.

Today some methods used by those schools have been incorporated into modern vision therapy, ways of correcting such disorders as failure of the two eyes to work together properly and training eye muscles to function more effectively.

For example, eye-training techniques can be applied to the vision of children with learning disabilities. A problem for some children who are otherwise quick and intelligent is an inability to copy on paper what they see on the classroom blackboard. The eye muscles they use to focus on the blackboard are too inefficient to shift the focus of the eyes to the paper. Vision therapy can be instituted to give the eye muscles exercise in shifting from far to near and back again. After about three months, the muscles are usually strong enough to function properly.

A myth about sight, persistent among many elderly people, is that using remaining vision will ruin it, a concept in vogue decades ago and even fostered by many eye doctors and therapists. The myth persists, especially among those who grew up with it. As one low vision specialist says, "Eyesight isn't something you can deposit in a savings account. It's something that should be invested and put to work."

Learning to see is a lifelong process, not one that ends in infancy. I discovered this for myself a few years ago. Every day on the way to my office in Washington, D.C., I passed without paying much attention to it an immense gray stone building on the corner of Pennsylvania Avenue and 17th Street. This massive edifice seemed extravagantly overdone in contrast to the breathtaking simplicity of the White House beside it. In a sense I punished its architectural flamboyance by ignoring it. On my first trip to Europe, I stood transfixed, listening to professional guides expound on the architectural excellencies of buildings that I realized (with a sort of cultural shame) were not one whit handsomer than that edifice I had disdained every day. On my return, I saw it as if for the first time, truly an architectural treasure, a historic landmark, the former War and Navy Building, now the Old Executive Office Building. With eyes newly educated by foreign guides, I discovered the beauties of this building, its carved lintels and graceful colonnades, the variety of ornament, and through the tall windows glimpses of splendid crystal chandeliers. I had learned to see with appreciation.

In the human eye, cones—closely packed cells in the retina directly behind the lens—control central, sharply focused vision and color vision. Rods respond to signals from the periphery, enabling us to see areas beyond the central vision. Some animals have only rod cells, others—some birds, for instance, high-flying predators—have only cones, which seem to be all they need for pinpointing prey on the ground. Hawks can spot a mouse as much as a half mile below them.

While doing a spectacular job on the adaptive visual systems of other creatures, nature seems to have been shortsighted about the demands that civilization would make on human eyes. To be sure, nature supplied us with a bifocal system that enables our two eyes to view objects straight in front of us without our being obliged, like birds, to turn our heads, and it supplied us with a generous supply of rods in the retina to help us encompass vistas and to see at night.

But nature's prescience about the needs of mankind in a literate, industrialized world faltered about the time the printing press made its debut in the fifteenth century. For the vision-demanding work of reading—and the subsequent work of operating fast-moving machines, driving cars and flying planes—nature provided a concentration of cones one-twentieth of an inch in diameter, respectfully dubbed the "Mighty Mac" by some eye researchers. In a diagram of the retina, the macula is a mere jog in the outline, as if someone had startled the graphic artist and jarred his hand. Yet, this tiny area is responsible for central vision essential for seeing details. The macula is especially prone to the onslaughts of aging; in low vision clinics macular degeneration is the most common disorder for which patients seek help.

Not being able to see an object though it's in plain sight, right in front of our eyes, is a common experience at any age, but it happens more frequently as we get older, and memory, an essential element in vision, loses some of its keenness. I remarked to a friend that one of the most exasperating experiences was to go into a room to get something, being unable to remember what I was looking for, and being obliged to return to the room I came from to jog my memory. "You're lucky," my friend said. "I can't even remember what room I came from."

These lapses in visual memory, when what we're looking for may be in plain sight, are due to the intrusion of other thoughts while we're in transit. Determined one day not to be defeated by this lapse of memory that interfered with my seeing and resolved not to return to the room I had come from, I visualized my electronic calculator and mentally pressed the "clear" button. Standing motionless, I forced my brain to clear itself and become a blank. I could feel my shoulders relax and after a few moments free of distracting inputs, the visual image of the object I sought appeared as if by magic. This mental trick has worked ever since, not always instantly, to be sure—an exercise in improving memory and concentration. Such exercises are useful to those with normal vision and essential to the partially sighted, who must use their residual vision with maximum efficiency.

The visual-acuity rating in an eye examination applies only to the situation in which the examination takes place, the controlled conditions of the eye doctor's office. In the "real world" everyone's vision, no matter how keen, is impaired at some time or another by what you might call situational influences. As psychiatrist Karl Menninger points out in *The Human Mind,* "A man may be blinded with rage; a child may be too overwhelmed with anxiety to see or hear correctly." Though there may be no defect in the eyes themselves, emotional stress can throw the eye/brain visual system out of kilter, distorting or blotting out images altogether.

We are apt to consider the eyes as organs in some way separate from the influence of the body's physical condition, but they are in fact as sensitive as seismographs. Besides the effects just noted (rage and anxiety), the quality of vision is affected by the body's general health. Paralyzing strokes can cause blindness, usually in one eye. Such chronic diseases as diabetes and high blood pressure affect the eyes, and even temporary illnesses such as severe head colds and nausea can reduce our ability to see clearly. When the stress of fatigue becomes excessive, the eyes refuse to work any longer and lower their lids, obliging us to doze lightly or sleep deeply.

Our visual abilities decline when we are bored or distracted. In my childhood, what greeted us when we entered the public library was the sign on the librarian's desk: SILENCE. That printed admonition seemed to us just another officious adult rule. But some of us later on would understand its purpose. Silence enhances the visual efficiency of readers by helping them concentrate. This intangible aid to seeing is, I realize, not easy to achieve in libraries or homes these days. There may be some correlation between the semi-illiteracy among today's young people and the fact that they study with rock music blasting away in the background. But there's no doubt whatsoever that partially sighted family members could see better if the decibel level of hi-fi sets were lowered.

Curiously, motivation, the will to see—or not see—can affect the quality of vision. The truck driver with failing vision takes an eye examination in quite a different frame of mind from that of a person with good vision who goes for a regular eye checkup. The truck driver, his job possibly at stake, sharply focuses not only his eyes but his mind on the chart letters. He strives to see, leans forward, almost willing those letters into greater clarity. This "psychic concentration" often pays off in a higher acuity rating, though the results in that controlled setting bear little relation to how clearly he sees on the highway at two in the morning after driving his tractor-trailer hundreds of miles, his mind dulled with fatigue and boredom.

In contrast to that highly motivated truck driver is the aging typist, indifferent to her work, who hopes her deteriorating eyesight will qualify her for disability retirement. During the eye examination, she leans back, unconsciously distancing herself from the chart and only half-focuses her eyes on it. If the eye doctor, instead of certifying her for disability retirement, merely gives her a prescription for stronger glasses, she hates him.

Some patients who want eye doctors to certify them as legally blind in order to qualify for financial and other benefits, memorize the letters on the eye chart and during the eye examination deliberately misread them. According to eye doctors in low vision clinics, this type of "cheating" is rare, and rarely are they taken in by it. Quite different is the motivation of some elderly men and women who memorize the chart letters to impress the doctor with their "remarkable" vision for their age and win coveted praise. They leave the doctor's office still half-blind, but feeling good about themselves.

Does our visual system do more than receive beams of light and transform them into electrochemical signals to the brain, where they are interpreted? "The eyes converse as much as tongues," Ralph Waldo Emerson said, "and their ocular dialogue needs no dictionary, but is understood the world over." More than passive recorders, the eyes can be activists with powers of their own as we know from poets and painters and from our own experience. Stare at an unfriendly dog and it will most likely bark or attack. The power of the eyes to cause mischief by merely looking, the "evil eye," is feared in all cultures the world over. In some primitive societies, the eye of the camera acquires the power of a human eye that can "kidnap the soul."

The mysterious power of the eyes finds articulation among city dwellers in the "etiquette of looking"—staring is taboo. Waiting for elevators, people avoid each other's eyes, watch the elevator indicator, or withdraw into self-conscious detachment. In crowded elevators, buses, subways, passengers, though crushed together, accept the physical contact so long as there is no eye contact between them. It is a matter of visual territory, not to be breached by strangers.

Most of the time, except when performing a task, we see unconsciously, our minds engaged with other matters. But people with partial sight see with a purpose. "Unconscious viewing is not for them," says Dr. Economon. "People with partial sight generally use it more efficiently than those with normal vision. They have to work at seeing. They have to use special visual aids and, in some instances, learn to see in a different way, using peripheral vision as a substitute for lost central vision."

What many people with low vision don't realize, says Dr. Economon, "is that despite efforts of eye doctors and therapists to get the message over to them, they are surrounded by people with 20/20 visual acuity who get less out of their perfect vision than most people with impaired vision, who, obliged to see with a purpose, use what vision they have to better advantage."

It does not occur to people with normal vision to ask themselves what they want to see. Their minds select and their eyes comply. But the question, "What do you want to see?" is one of the first that patients in low vision clinics must answer. How they answer that question is the basis for the treatment program, including the selection of visual aids that will help them achieve their purpose. In a later chapter we'll go into how realistically most low vision patients answer the question: "What do you want to see?"

3

Major Causes of Low Vision Problems

Before considering some of the major eye disorders that plague Americans and cause impaired vision, we'll briefly review the eyes themselves, their parts, normal functions, and role in the eye/brain visual system.

No matter how healthy it is or how efficient its parts, without light, the eye cannot see anything. The first portal through which light enters the eye is the *cornea,* the crystalline part of the outer eye, a sort of organic contact lens covering the iris and pupil. The cornea serves not only as a conduit for light beams, but bends them, providing about 65 percent of the refractive power of the eye. There are no blood vessels in the cornea, a factor that contributes to its transparency and, it is believed, facilitates corneal transplants. The most sensitive tissue in the body, the cornea's seventy

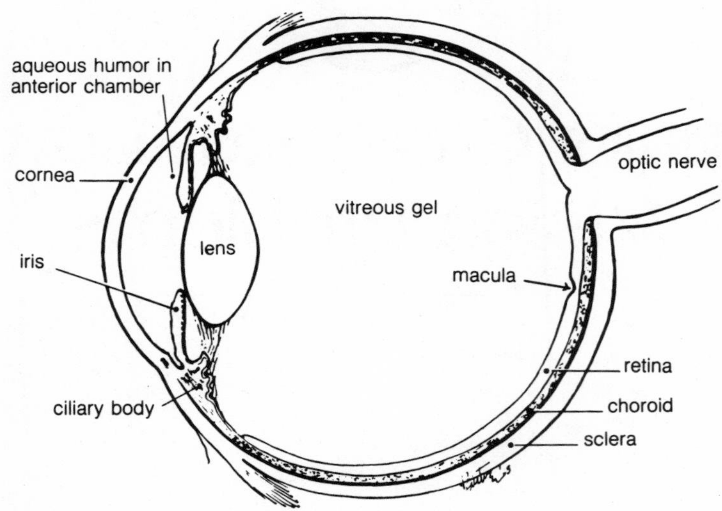

Diagram of the eye. (NATIONAL EYE INSTITUTE)

naked nerve fibers account for the intense pain caused by even tiny particles, chemical or other burns, or wounds.

Just behind the cornea is a space called the anterior chamber, which houses the *aqueous humor,* a watery fluid continuously produced and continuously drained away. Manufactured by the *ciliary body* (see below), this fluid supplies nutrients to and removes waste products from the back surface of the cornea and lens.

The *pupil,* which looks like a flat black disk, is actually the window to the eye's interior. Before the invention of the ophthalmoscope, eye doctors could not see through that window into the dark interior of the eye.

Surrounding the pupil is the *iris,* the colored part of the eye that, by contracting or expanding the size of the pupil, controls the amount of light entering the eye.

Light makes its way to the *lens,* a transparent structure that has no blood vessels or nerves. Suspended behind the iris, the lens focuses light on the retina. A healthy lens in young people is colorless, but with age it becomes yellowish, loses its elasticity and some of its ability to adjust itself to focus on near and distant objects. When an opacity, called a cataract, forms in the lens, it blocks the passage of light, causing loss of central vision.

The *ciliary* body, besides secreting aqueous fluid, helps provide muscular control of the lens.

Like air in a football, the *vitreous,* a clear, gelatinous body, maintains the shape of the eye. Without the vitreous, the eye would collapse. During vitrectomy (surgery to correct defects in the vitreous) a saline solution simultaneously replaces the vitreous fluid being withdrawn.

The tough outer coating enclosing the eyeball, except for the cornea, is the whitish *sclera,* sometimes tinged with blue in Caucasians, slightly yellowish in the eyes of Orientals and Blacks. Its highly polished surface contributes much to the beauty of human and animal eyes. But it has a practical function too—its toughness protects the delicate interior structures of the eyes.

Covering the sclera is the *conjunctiva,* a thin, transparent membrane that also lines the inside of the eyelids. Besides being a protective coating, it helps keep the cornea moist. Nourished by many blood vessels, it has, however, few pain fibers, and therefore even major inflammations of the conjunctiva rarely cause pain.

Between the sclera and the retina is a layer of tissue, the *choroid,* rich in blood vessels that carry a nourishing blood supply to the eyes.

Lining the inside back part of the eye is the *retina,* a thin, delicate light-sensitive membrane, the only visible part of the brain outside the skull. Composed of layers of cells called rods and cones, the retina responds to visual stimuli by a photochemical action. The photoreceptive rods and cones convert incoming light into electrical signals that are processed and integrated into an exquisitely organized cellular system in the brain. Rods predominate in the periphery of the retina, providing side and up-and-down vision (*where* vision) in natural or artificial light, but their main job is to help us see at night. Cones are packed into the *macula,* that 1/20-inch area in the retina that gives us sharp detailed vision (*what* vision) for reading and other close work and for seeing things straight ahead. Cones are also the regulators of color perception.

The photochemical signals from the retina are transmitted to visual centers of the brain by the *optic nerves,* cables of numerous nerve fibers. If the optic nerves are damaged by injury or atrophy, sight is generally lost. Repair of optic nerves is an area of visual research that so far has not yielded solutions, but studies in nerve regeneration, one of the most active research areas in biology, give hope that scientists may one day come up with a way of restoring function to damaged optic nerves.

To follow through on this minitour of the eyes, the cells in the optic nerve and optic tract connect with a group of cells in the thalamus of the brain. From there, nerve impulses go to an area of the visual cortex at the back of the brain and there, electrochemical messages are decoded and transformed into images.

Before completing our tour of the eye, we should mention two other practical, ingenious devices that protect them—eyelids and eyelashes. The movement of the lids is so rapid that we are unaware of it. It is estimated that, during a lifetime, the lids go up and down about a quarter of a billion times. Their efficiency, however, can be impaired by fatigue and drugs, including alcohol.

Eyelashes serve as screens to protect the eyes from dust and other particles. They also serve an aesthetic purpose by accentuating the beauty of the eyes with a natural outline and by casting a subtle shadow on them to give them depth. Since ancient times, women have sought to improve on nature by using eyeliners—kohl in ancient Egypt, and today various colored eye pencils and mascara, even false eyelashes. But try as they may, women cannot rival the most luxuriant eyelashes in the world—the eyelashes of the camel. Not that they do much to improve the camel's looks, but they do help keep the sand out of the animal's eyes.

With some understanding of the infinite complexity of the anatomy of the eyes, you may have an inkling that things can go wrong with parts of this remarkable apparatus. Not that everyone has considered the eye remarkable. The great nineteenth-century ophthalmologist, Hermann von Helmholtz, is reported to have remarked that if an optical instrument maker offered him the eye as an optical apparatus, he would have rejected it out of hand because of the carelessness of its construction. Helmholtz devised the ophthalmoscope, but he never came up with a better eye.

Only eye-care practitioners need to know all the disorders that afflict the eyes. But a small number of disorders account for the majority of eye impairments. The most prevalent disorders affecting millions of Americans are cataracts, glaucoma, retinal and corneal disorders, and congenital diseases.

Cataracts

"If we live long enough, we'll all have them," one ophthalmologist gloomily predicts, and another puts it more specifically: "Of those of us who survive into our seventies, one in four will have cataracts."

Fifty years ago that would have been frightening news indeed. As Dr. Jules Stein, one of the great figures in vision research, told an audience on the occasion of his acceptance of the Albert Lasker Public Service Award:

> When I left the practice of ophthalmology in 1925, a cataract operation was an extremely dangerous procedure.

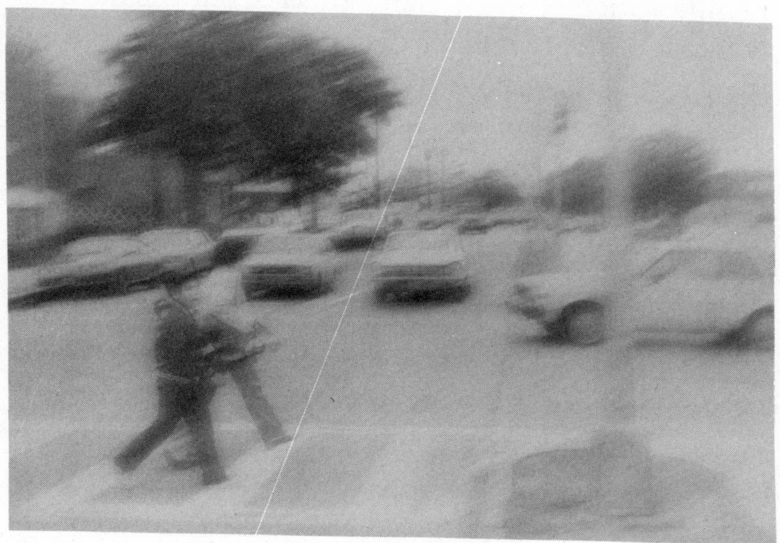

Cataracts: A clouding of the lens that causes a general loss of detail in what a person sees. The field of vision is unaffected, but glaring light conditions, distortion and double images can prove annoying.
(AMERICAN FOUNDATION FOR THE BLIND)

We broke up the lens with a needle and scratched out whatever part of it we could reach. Patients were immobilized for weeks, their heads between sandbags. If they were lucky enough to avoid postoperative infections that might have destroyed their sight, they were required to wear beer-bottle lenses that not only were ugly, but distorted the world around them.

Cataracts—a leading cause of blindness in the United States—occur most frequently in the elderly, a manifestation of aging, like wrinkles, but the disorder is found not only among the elderly; some babies are born with cataracts or develop them within the first year of life. Some of these congenital cataracts are due to faulty genes; others result from infections such as German measles (rubella) contracted by the mother during pregnancy. Before inoculations against German measles became an accepted public-health measure, thousands of babies whose mothers had been infected with rubella were born blind.

Cataracts can occur at any age from a variety of causes: prenatal infections, injuries to the eyes from blows to the head and exposure to certain chemicals and radiation. Some drugs, most commonly cortisone and its derivatives, used to treat systemic diseases may induce cataracts. Physicians and patients faced with the harrowing choice must weigh the gravity of the disease being treated against the risk of inducing cataracts. Intense heat from prolonged exposure to blast furnaces or to desert sunlight can also cause a clouding of the lens with consequent loss of vision. And some metabolic disorders such as diabetes may contribute to the formation of cataracts.

Sixty percent of cataracts occur in people between sixty-five and seventy-four years of age. It is predictable that as the number of elderly increases, so will the incidence of cataracts. This disorder is not confined to industrial nations. According to the World Health Organization (WHO), in developing countries cataracts are a major cause of avoidable blindness, occurring in some seventeen million people.

Today's cataract operations are considered by ophthalmic surgeons to be 95 percent successful. This is due to improved surgical techniques and advances in instrumentation. Biomedical engineers have worked hand in glove, so to speak, with surgeons, developing scissors so small they could fit within the circumference of a dime and sutures finer than human hair. Equally important are the electronic optical aids that highly magnify and thus enable surgeons to see parts of the eye that formerly they could only guess at.

An advance of incalculable significance in the evolution of cataract surgery was the development of the plastic lens to replace the natural, defective lens at the time of its removal. Termed an intraocular lens, its use was approved for marketing in 1981 by the Food and Drug Administration (FDA) following years of experimental use during which the plastic lenses were demonstrated to be safe and effective. Of the one million cataract operations performed in the United States in 1985, an estimated 85 percent involved the implantation of intraocular lenses, now considered one of the safest and most effective major surgical procedures.

No one knows how effective these implants will be over a period of twenty or more years. Cautious about the longevity of these implants, many physicians do not advocate their being used in younger people who, after cataract surgery, have alternative types of lenses (prescription eyeglasses or contact lenses) to replace a surgically removed lens.

Research in pediatric surgery, including a better understanding of anesthesia for infants, has made possible eye operations on babies only a few weeks old. Dr. David Schaffer, director of the division of ophthalmology at Children's Hospital in Philadelphia, which pioneered the use of soft contact lenses in infants after removal of cataracts, says, "Without a lens, the baby's eyes cannot focus, so an artificial means must be substituted for the surgically removed lens. It's extremely important that the infant spend a minimum amount of time without lenses."

Though rare, congenital cataracts account for 11.5 percent of blindness in preschool children. Signs of cataracts in infants include an obvious white spot on the pupil, crossed eyes (strabismus), or an unnaturally rapid movement of the eyes (nystagmus). Any of these symptoms should prompt parents to take the baby to an eye doctor for early diagnosis and treatment. One point that pediatric ophthalmologists emphasize is early correction of visual defects in infants, essential if the visual system is to develop properly.

At the other end of the age scale are heartening reports of elderly men and women seeing after a lifetime of blindness. One grandmother in her seventies saw her children and grandchildren for the first time after cataract surgery. Her great regret was that the husband to whom she had been married for forty-six years had died nine years before the sight-giving surgery that would have enabled her to see him.

Not every cataract is a candidate for removal. If the opacity does not interfere with reading or driving or other habitual activities, vision improvement after the removal of a cataract is unlikely to match the patient's expectations. There will not only be disappointment, but a sense of letdown, even transitory depression. As Dr. Julius Shulman says in his book, *Cataracts,* "A cataract does not have to be removed just because it's there." The criterion Dr. Shulman gives for cataract surgery is "when you can no longer see well enough to do the things you enjoy, perform your daily activities in a satisfactory manner and function adequately and happily."

When impaired vision results from several factors, not solely a cataract, removing the cataract may not solve the total vision problem. A person who has glaucoma, for example, may have to postpone cataract surgery until the glaucoma can be controlled. Retinal disorders such as fissures put patients at high risk of exacerbating the retinal condition by cataract surgery. Though people with diabetes have good prospects for successful cataract surgery, they too are at somewhat higher risk because of possible damage to the eyes caused by the diabetes. Fearful of failure and discomfort, many elderly people have refused cataract surgery, but as reports of the phenomenal success of this type of surgery have circulated, thousands of fearful elderly men and women have pushed aside their apprehensions and opted for surgery.

The number of cataract operations performed in the United States each year is likely to increase apace with the growing number of elderly people. Eye surgery, once rare and risky, as techniques and knowledge of the eyes advance, is attracting young ophthalmologists in greater numbers, and as more ophthalmologists are trained in cataract surgery and become experienced in the technique, the higher will be the level of proficiency.

But what most concerns us in this book is the fact that, of the one million cataract operations performed each year, about 5 percent, affecting some 50,000 men, women and children, are considered failures—that is, the eyesight of these patients is not improved and in some cases is worsened, because of postoperative complications. Hemorrhaging in one or both eyes, retinal fissures, opacities that occur when the lens casing is left to form a buffer, an implanted lens that for some reason fails to give clear vision—these are some of the reasons for cataract surgical failures.

Low vision clinics are dealing with many of these failed cataract operations. Dr. H. MacKenzie Freeman, senior clinical scientist and vice-president of the Eye Research Institute of the Retina Foundation, in Boston, told participants in a low vision symposium that in many cases new surgical procedures are used on patients with eye conditions so severe that treatment, no matter how successful, improves vision only up to the low vision range. Surgical treatment can take these patients only so far. Where surgical treatment ends, he said, low vision evaluation should begin. This next step in the continuum of eye care involves a comprehensive study of retinal function, a low vision assessment to determine visual needs and desires, followed by the prescription of low vision aids, then mobility training and counseling on social adjustment.

The Retina

On a day in May 1943, Hector Chevigny, a successful author and scriptwriter in his early forties, was walking on Hollywood's Vine Street when, as he described it in his book *My Eyes Have a Cold Nose,* from the upper-left corner of his field of vision "a jet black curtain descended, stopping just short of the median line and cutting across the field diagonally. There was not only no pain, there was no sensation whatsoever. Half my retina had torn loose from its moorings, as I found when I could get to an ophthalmologist. A few hours later the retina completed its detachment." Hector was blind in one eye.

As a boy he had developed "juvenile cataracts," which had been successfully removed. But at that time no one warned him that removal of cataracts might put him at risk for possible retinal detachment later on. When the detachment occurred, doctors decided against trying to repair the retina in an eye somewhat atrophied by disease. Not especially concerned about having only one good eye, Hector traveled by train from California to New York to a new job, a cross-country trip that in the 1940s took several days and subjected passengers to considerable jolting.

A week after his arrival in New York, the retina in

his good eye began to tear away. The eye doctor who, like all his colleagues not in military service during the war, had more patients than he could manage effectively, advised Hector to return at once to California where his wife, Claire, and their two children were waiting for him to get settled in New York. Hector realized this was not good advice, especially after that long, jolting train ride across the country. Traveling by air was out of the question for ordinary civilians during

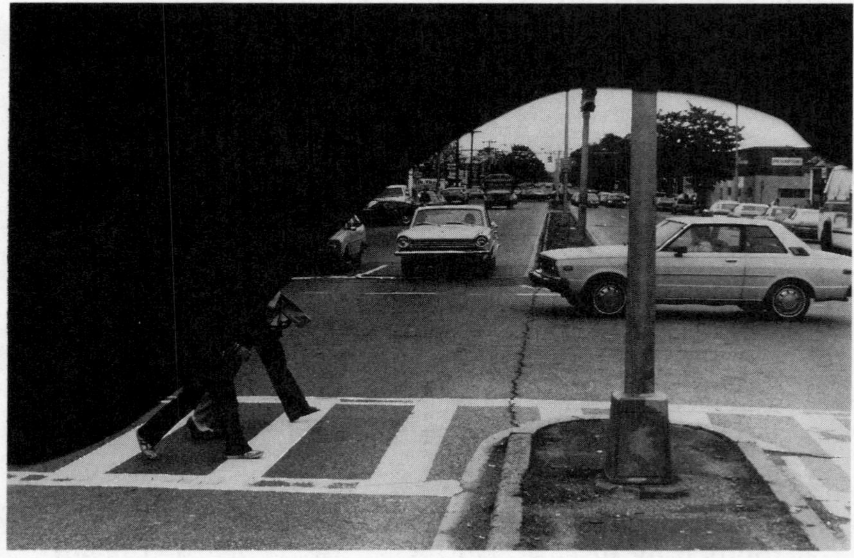

Detached Retina: Retinas detach for a variety of reasons, and many can be surgically repaired. When active, the hole or tear fills with fluid, lifting the retina from its normal position and causing a defect in the field of vision. These defects can appear as dark shadows, either above or below the central field, as though a hanging curtain or wave was obstructing vision. (AMERICAN FOUNDATION FOR THE BLIND)

wartime. Hector, through friends, found another doctor in New York who ordered him into the hospital immediately. But, unable to accept the prognosis of the second retinal detachment, Hector refused to go. Several days after seeing that doctor, the retina detached. It was, as he describes it in his book, "as if an invisible finger had pushed down my retina and crumpled it halfway, as it would a piece of cellophane. My vision clouded past the center. Accompanying the drop was a startling display of bright-blue fireworks, like the northern borealis at its brightest. Queerly, I was suddenly calm."

When I first met Hector, he had been blind for several years. He, Claire, and their two children, and Hector's seeing-eye dog, a magnificent boxer named Wizard (the "cold nose" in the title of Hector's book), were neighbors of mine in New York. During the many walks Hector, Wizard and I took in a nearby park, Hector talked about those months in the hospital and the three unsuccessful attempts to reattach the retinas of both eyes. For weeks he had to lie perfectly still, his head between sandbags, an ordeal for anyone, but for a nervous, impatient man almost impossible. Not only did I learn about how a man coped with blindness on a high-pressure job and getting about New York with a guide dog, but I got from Hector an insight into the blindness establishment, which he believed was anachronistic. Years later when I read his book, I realized that on those walks through the park he was composing the first draft of the book.

Though surgical repair of detached retinas has been

practiced since 1929, the success rate even at the time of Hector's unsuccessful surgery in 1943 was low. Surgeons used traditional instruments—scalpel, needle and thread. They did not have the powerful magnifying electronic microscopes of today. New types of instruments, materials and techniques, even the ingenious upside-down operating table that uses gravity as an aid in repairing detached retinas have increased the rate of success and decreased the length of time a patient spends in the hospital.

Retinal detachments can be caused by a shrinkage of the vitreous gel and the consequent pull on the retina, tearing it away from the back of the eye. Most commonly, retinal detachment is associated with retinal breaks, tiny defects in the fragile membrane, or diseases such as diabetes that damage the eyes. Injuries to the head or eyes are another cause of detached retinas, a fact commonly occurring among professional boxers as was the case most recently with Sugar Ray Leonard.

Others who run the risk of retinal detachment are those who have had "juvenile cataracts" removed, as was undoubtedly the case with Hector Chevigny, which is one important reason for follow-up after cataract surgery. Certain types of myopia or nearsightedness that run in families often, in combination with other optical defects, can result in retinal detachments.

Laser surgery, first widely used in the 1970s, marked a milestone in the treatment of eye disorders, including retinal detachments. Instead of cutting into an eye with a scalpel, the surgeon uses a laser, split-second bursts of intense light focused through the pupil to a particular spot on the retina. The patient sits opposite the laser specialist and, head held steady by clamps, looks straight ahead as the laser beam is focused on the precise spot in the retina that is to receive the intense light.

Cryotherapy is another technique used in retinal

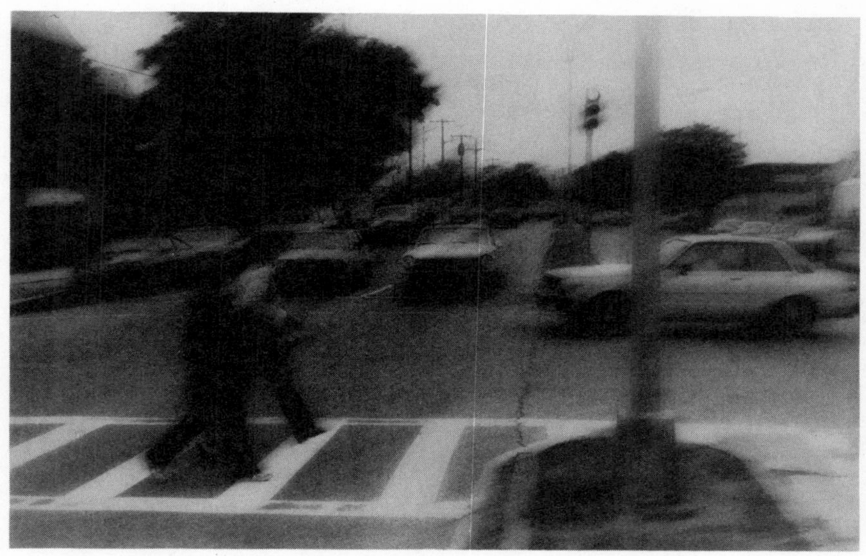

Diabetic Retinopathy: About 80 percent of diabetics with this disease experience, at most, a swelling and leaking of retinal blood vessels, which may cause blurring of the central field. The balance of cases develop into a proliferative state, interfering with light passage through the eye —either in random patterns or throughout the visual field. Most commonly, some vision remains intact.
(AMERICAN FOUNDATION FOR THE BLIND)

surgery. In cryotherapy the surgeon freezes a retinal hole to promote the growth of sealing scar tissue. The sooner such holes are detected, the more effectively treatment can seal them and prevent their turning into large tears that can lead to retinal detachment.

Diabetic retinopathy, the principal cause of new blindness in the United States, is another retinal disorder. This disease attacks the retinas of those who have had diabetes for many years. But because it is a threat to every diabetic, doctors urge diabetics to have their eyes tested every six months.

Characteristic of diabetic retinopathy is the proliferation of "rogue" blood vessels in the retina and vitreous. These new blood vessels, less sturdy than normal ones, tend to break and leak blood that clouds the eye and obstructs the passage of light. Not too many years ago, medical scientists discovered the laser technique for sealing those leaking blood vessels, another marker in eye-treatment advances of the last decade. But though early detection of the leaking vessels enables treatment by photocoagulation, there is so far no way of preventing the formation of new rogue blood vessels. That's why vigilance on the part of patients and their eye doctors is essential to control those vessels in their early stages.

Control of diabetic retinopathy cannot be separated from control of diabetes itself, of which the eye disorder is a pernicious side effect. Some ten million Americans have diabetes, now considered by medical scientists to be not one but several diseases. The two major types of diabetes are the early-onset type, a congenital disorder that occurs in young people, and the more common adult-onset type, which develops in middle and later years. Until the discovery of insulin in 1921 by two Canadian researchers, Frederick G. Banting and Charles H. Best, one of the great scientific achievements of the twentieth century, diabetes was an incurable, usually fatal disease.

Not all diabetics need insulin treatment: millions control the disease by special diets, exercise, and abstaining from alcohol and cigarettes. But an estimated one million Americans, young and old, depend on injected or orally administered insulin for survival. This life-saving drug has been found to be not so benign as at first believed. For those who have been taking it for years, it has been the cause of heart attacks, strokes, kidney failure, gangrene and blindness.

Though insulin saves the lives of diabetics, it cannot prevent serious complications of the disease. There is no way of predicting what some of those complications may be, but one thing is certain: the eyes are likely targets of the disease. According to the American Foundation for the Blind, diabetes is the major cause of new blindness each year in the United States. Much of this could be prevented by early detection and control of the disease itself. Once the disease is diagnosed, patients must cooperate fully in treatments, and, if they want to prolong healthy eyesight, should have twice-yearly eye exams. Failure to adhere to the demands of the regimen is often a matter of economics, according to Theresa Travis, supervisor of rehabilitation at the Columbia Lighthouse for the Blind in Washington, D.C.

> For one person in a poor family to follow a special diet is often financially impossible. The rest of the family may want entirely different meals from what the person with diabetes is obliged to eat and purchasing small quantities of special foods is usually much more expensive than buying large quantities for a big family. Physicians don't always take this into account when prescribing special diets. Nor do some eye doctors realize that poor patients who have trouble scraping up round-trip bus fares are often unable to make frequent visits to the doctor's office for eye checkups. The sound advice given by doctors and recommended in health pamphlets is often disregarded by diabetics, not from indifference, but because poor patients can't afford to follow it.

Macular Degeneration

Someone I know recalls this episode: she had never heard the term "macular degeneration" until, at the end of a routine eye examination, the doctor said matter-of-factly: "You're going blind. You have senile macular degeneration."

Actually, she did not hear the term then. Her mind had clamped down on the word *blind.* It was only a few days later, after she had partially recovered from the shock and had called the doctor to find out what he had said was the cause of her inevitable blindness, that she heard clearly and unforgettably the words "senile macular degeneration." *Senile!* And she wasn't even sixty-five yet. In moments of deep depression she considered suicide. But turning away from that route, she went to another ophthalmologist, who examined her eyes, said there were signs of deterioration in the macula of one eye, but the other looked healthy and would probably not show signs of deterioration for years. In any case, this eye doctor assured her she would not go blind even though she might eventually lose central vision in both eyes. There were low vision aids that, along with learning to see in a different way (eccentric viewing) using the peripheral cells in the retina, would enable her to read, keep her job, and live a normal life. She was one of the lucky ones who had found an eye doctor who knew the difference between blindness and partial sight, and who knew what could be done with functional vision.

The term *senile macular degeneration* is deplored by many eye doctors. Dr. J. Donald Gass of the Bascom Palmer Eye Institute at the Miami University School of Medicine, says:

> The term "macular degeneration" refers to a group of diseases that selectively cause deterioration of the retina in the macula region. One of the most common diseases is called "macular degeneration associated with drusen," or more frequently by the inappropriate name "senile macular degeneration." The name is inappropriate, firstly, because although most patients experience loss of vision when fifty years or older, some do so at a younger

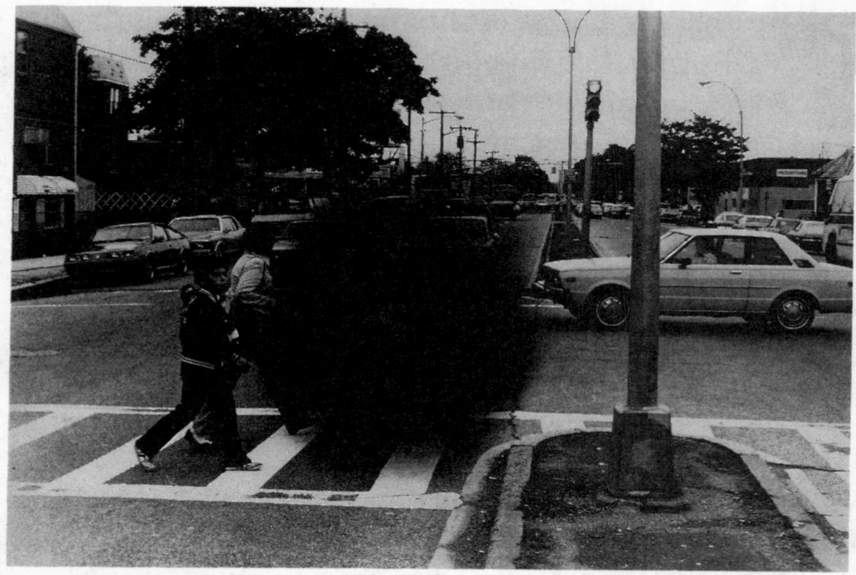

Macular Degeneration: The most common eye disease, macular degeneration, causes loss of vision in the central field, making it difficult to read or do close work. Remaining side vision makes object detection possible.
(AMERICAN FOUNDATION FOR THE BLIND)

age. Secondly, the name "senile" suggests that the patient's disease may be caused by arteriosclerosis (hardening of the arteries) and that he or she has necessarily lost other physical or mental faculties. The disease usually occurs in patients in good health. It is not caused by arteriosclerosis, nor is it related to any other medical disease, such as high blood pressure and diabetes, or to environmental factors, such as dietary deficiency, exposure to the sun, overuse of the eyes, smoking, or drinking alcoholic beverages. This form of macular degeneration is a deterioration that affects only the small part of the retina called the "macula" and is probably caused by an abnormality in the patient's genetic make-up.

If you may recall from our minitour of the eye, the macula is that tiny area in the retina responsible for our sharp, detailed vision. Disorders of the macula usually result from a proliferation of new blood vessels in the retina from unknown causes or from injuries to the eyes or to the head, or from some defect in the genes. An unusual case of damage to the macula occurred in a fifteen-year-old girl who, despite warnings in the media, watched an eclipse of the sun for ninety minutes. The next day, she noticed a loss of vision. The ophthalmologist who examined her eyes found that the intense light she had been staring at had burned the macula. She lost 75 percent of the vision in her left eye and 50 percent in the right eye, sight losses that were irreversible.

The two major types of macular disorders are those that are inherited and those that develop in the later years. The inherited type, generally referred to as "juvenile macular degeneration," begins before the age of twenty and severely handicaps students in their studies and limits their career choices. It's a rare but destructive disease for which there is no cure. But in this era of low vision services, identification of usable areas of the retina in combination with custom-designed aids and training in eccentric viewing, plus recorded texts and other books, "talking" computers, and the Kurzweil Reading Machine enable these young people to keep up with sighted classmates and open up a range of business and professional careers that thirty years ago would have been closed to them.

To get an idea of how vision is affected by macular degeneration, put a dab of toothpaste or shaving cream (about a quarter of an inch) on your eyeglass lens directly in front of the pupil, or, if you don't wear eyeglasses, put the dab on a piece of clear plastic and hold it up to one eye. Close the other eye and look straight ahead at the dab. You can't see through that quarter-inch obstruction; your central vision is blocked. That's what happens when the macula is impaired. But chances are you can see the area surrounding the obstruction; your peripheral vision is working. Would you consider yourself blind with all that functional vision going for you even though you couldn't see objects directly in front of you? In most instances of macular degeneration, peripheral vision works well. Lack of focal vision doesn't mean that a person is blind, but many eye specialists equate the inability to read eye charts with blindness.

According to Dr. Michael Wolffe, senior lecturer in the University of Aston's Department of Ophthalmic Optics in England, standard distance visual-acuity tests provide information about something *less than one percent* of the visual field. "Whilst this central one percent of vision is of paramount importance in terms of the recognition of fine detail, it is virtually useless in the absence of the rest of the visual field. It is the surrounding field of vision which, whilst not providing critical definition, is critical in terms of the location and detection of objects in the first place." In most instances of macular degeneration, peripheral vision remains intact and modern optics and training in the use of peripheral vision compensate for the loss of central vision, putting the patient in the category of the partially sighted, not of the blind.

Senile macular degeneration (SMD) affects some 670,000 Americans over sixty-five years of age, including 10 percent of those over seventy. The exact cause is unknown, but some medical scientists think it may result from a breakdown in the blood supply to the retina. A characteristic of the disorder, similar to diabetic retinopathy, is the formation of new fragile blood vessels in the choroid underlying the retina. These abnormal vessels are apt to break and leak into the macula, destroying healthy cells and causing loss of vision in that central area of tightly packed cones that enable us to see in clear detail whatever we focus our eyes on.

To find out if something could be done to arrest the development of SMD, the National Eye Institute launched a five-year study of the disorder. In 1982, three years into the study, the Institute announced dramatic findings from the twelve medical centers participating in the study. Calling the findings a giant step in combatting visual loss from SMD, the Institute reported that, if applied early enough in the development of the disease, photocoagulation using lasers could seal the abnormal blood vessels and prevent leakage into the macula. Photocoagulation, already used successfully in treating diabetic retinopathy, now began to be used in treating macular degeneration. But to be effective the laser treatment must be applied almost at the onset of SMD.

The study showed that if this type of macular disorder is not discovered in its early stages, the affected eye stands a 73 percent chance of losing some sight within a year and a half, and a 60 percent chance of suffering severe visual loss. There is a 42 percent chance the patient will become legally blind—that is, reach a visual acuity of 20/200 or less. Appropriately timed laser treatment, says the study report, can prevent or delay significantly 89 percent of the cases of severe visual impairment.

Unfortunately, even though SMD may be detected early, photocoagulation of the abnormal new blood vessels may not be possible if the vessels are too close to the center of the macula or are hidden from the laser surgeon's view by an infusion of blood.

How can you detect those subtle, telltale changes in your vision that could signal the onset of SMD without spending an inordinate amount of time going to a doctor's office? If you are forty-five or over, an annual eye exam is a must. Between eye examinations, if you suspect your vision is deteriorating, you can test it on what is called an Amsler grid. All ophthalmologists have copies of this grid, but you can easily make one. It is a piece of paper on which are printed vertical and horizontal lines, intersecting to form squares about the size of those in crossword puzzles. In the center of this grid is a black dot. Covering one eye, look at that dot. If there are blank areas around it or if the surrounding lines look bent or wavy, you could have trouble in your macula. It would be wise to see your eye doctor quickly.

Dr. Paul B. Freeman, specialist in low vision and director of the Center for Vision Rehabilitation in Aliquippa, Pennsylvania, says that advanced optical aids and special viewing techniques can help 90 to 95 percent of those who have macular degeneration. At the 1984 convention of the American Optometric Association, Dr. Freeman demonstrated some of those aids to the press. Among reporters present was Robert Trumbull of *The New York Times.* Trumbull, according to his own account, had "struggled" with macular degeneration for eight years only to be told by one eye doctor after another, "Nothing can be done." At Dr. Freeman's press conference, Trumbull took part in the demonstration. Recounting his experience in the *Times,* Trumbull wrote:

> Dr. Freeman moved one of the hotel's ordinary floor lamps to a spot beside this reporter's chair, so that light fell on the small optical chart in his hands, then clipped a pair of special lenses over the reporter's eyeglasses and directed him to look at the chart at various distances. At the ideal distance, using the badly damaged left eye alone and looking slightly to the right of the reprinted letters, the reporter read all the way down to the next to the last line, giving up on the final one, which was in the tiny print known in the trade as Bible type.

Like so many people with macular degeneration who have lost central vision in one eye, Trumbull had been concerned about being able to read and do his job as a reporter if he lost the sight of his "good eye." He came out of Dr. Freeman's demonstration a man freed from nagging anxiety and equipped to cope with his macular disorder.

In treating patients with macular degeneration, Dr. Freeman, like other low vision specialists, draws on an array of optical and nonoptical aids, including microscopes mounted in spectacle frames for reading and other close work, tiny telescopes inserted into conventional spectacle lenses for distance viewing, and telescopic lenses for typing and working with video display terminals. Patients select the aids best suited to their needs, and Dr. Freeman or his assistant gives them, along with their aids, the required training in their use and in off-center viewing.

Dr. DeWitt Stetten, Jr., Senior Science Advisor at the National Institutes of Health, in his article "Coping with Blindness," published in the *New England Journal of Medicine,* chided ophthalmologists for their disregard for the quality of life of a person whose vision is declining.

Dr. Stetten first learned that he had macular degeneration in the 1960s. He says in his article that in the fifteen years following the diagnosis, despite

> many contacts with skilled and experienced professionals, no ophthalmologist has at any time suggested any

device that might be of assistance to me. No ophthalmologist has mentioned any of the ways in which I could stem the deterioration in the quality of my life. Fortunately, I have discovered a number of means whereby I have helped myself, and the purpose of this essay is to call the attention of the ophthalmological world to some of these devices and, courteously but firmly, to complain of what appears to be the ophthalmologists' attitude: "We are interested in vision but have little interest in blindness."

Dr. Stetten went on to describe some of the devices that have helped him through the period of gradually declining sight, during which he carried on his NIH administrative duties as an institute director and later as Senior Science Advisor. While he had residual vision, he used a Visualtek machine that greatly magnified printed and typed materials. When he could no longer see, he discovered the Talking Books Program of the Library of Congress, obtained technical journals through Recorded Periodicals Services, and obtained a Kurzweil Reading Machine that enabled him to select books and periodicals he wanted to read and to "hear" his correspondence. Dr. Stetten told me that his most useful aids were a talking watch, a Norelco model miniature tape recorder he could hold in the palm of his hand or carry in his pocket, and an auto-dialer telephone with a memory that stores thirty-two phone numbers that he can dial merely by pressing one button.

Dr. Stetten remarked ruefully during our interview, "Eye specialists are more concerned with the eyeballs than with the person behind them." His article in the *New England Journal of Medicine* engendered a tremendous response from eye-care professionals, especially young ophthalmologists, and from physicians who had had similar experiences with their eye doctors. The article did much to educate ophthalmologists about their responsibilities to patients.

Glaucoma

To cataracts, diabetic retinopathy and macular degeneration, we must add the fourth major cause of severe vision impairment, including blindness: *glaucoma.* What sets this disorder apart from the other three is that it can be controlled and, if detected early, can be prevented from worsening by medications and in some instances by surgery. What is truly tragic is that, though it can be detected and treated, millions of Americans are unaware that they have the disorder and do not understand its terrible consequences. If glaucoma is not controlled, it can eventually destroy the optic nerve and when that happens, visual signals cannot be transmitted to the brain.

In 90 percent of cases, the onset is insidious. Glaucoma, called the "sneak thief of sight," is caused by a malfunction in the eye's remarkable drainage system: The ciliary body produces fluid that supplies nutrients and oxygen to the cornea and lens while simultaneously removing wastes from those tissues. This fluid keeps pressure within the eye higher than that of the

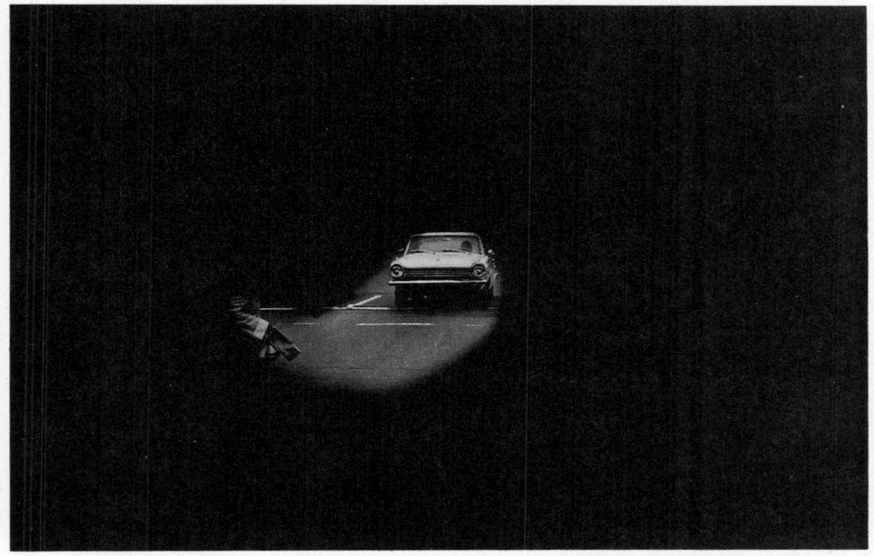

Glaucoma: A disease in which tissues are damaged by increasing pressure within the eye. If not treated soon enough, glaucoma can destroy side vision, leaving tunnel vision—a small central area in which a person sees.
(AMERICAN FOUNDATION FOR THE BLIND)

outside atmosphere so the eye doesn't collapse. But when the drainage system gets clogged or the fluid drains too slowly, pressure builds up in the eyes, causing damage ranging from a slight vision loss to total blindness.

The disorder is so highly individualistic that treatment, whether medication or surgery or both, must be specifically tailored to each patient's condition. A disconcerting characteristic of the disease is that pressure within the eye due to changes in the rate of aqueous-humor formation, fluctuates during the day, usually high in the morning and throughout the day, then declining during sleep at night.

Of the three major types of glaucoma, the most prevalent is called *chronic open-angle glaucoma;* it develops gradually over the years. Because there is no warning pain or other discomfort as blockage of normal fluid drainage causes pressure to rise in the eye, glaucoma steadily erodes peripheral vision, gradually constricting sight to a narrow opening, and eventually destroying the optic nerve.

Its inexorable progress can be halted, provided that it is detected in the early stages. Surgery, perforations in the iris to reduce the abnormal pressure, may be necessary, but in most instances, glaucoma is controlled by medication, usually eye drops. Some patients, especially the elderly and those with hand tremors who have difficulty putting drops into their eyes, may take the medication in pill form. Patients with glaucoma, like insulin-dependent diabetics, must adhere faithfully to the schedule for administering the medication.

Acute angle-closure glaucoma is a sudden, inexplicable rise in pressure in the eye. The acute attack is characterized by rapid loss of sight and severe, throbbing pain in the eye. The nausea and vomiting that commonly accompanies the attack might be mistaken for an acute gastrointestinal attack, except for the rapid loss of sight.

Acute angle-closure is a medical emergency that, unless treated within a matter of hours, can lead to irreversible loss of vision. During the acute phase, a doctor administers medications to halt the attack and to reduce the excessive pressure. In some instances, surgery may be necessary to correct the faulty drainage system. Fortunately, this type of glaucoma is rare, but it is an extremely dangerous threat to eyesight.

Congenital glaucoma, also rare, but devastating, may be present in the fetus or show up after the baby is born. A defect in the region of the angle formed by the iris and the cornea obstructs the outflow of the aqueous humor, causing chronically high pressure in the eye. One of the more obvious signs of the disorder in babies is considerably enlarged eyeballs. Also, the cornea may have a milky appearance. The pupil is large and fixed. Other signs are watery eyes when the baby isn't crying, convulsive blinking of the eyelids, and an abnormal sensitivity to bright light. These symptoms in their newborn babies should prompt parents to take them to an eye specialist.

Besides these primary types of glaucoma are those "secondary" glaucomas resulting from other eye disorders, such as inflammation of the uvea (comprising the iris, ciliary body and choroid), injuries, certain medications or eye surgery itself. The underlying cause of secondary glaucomas must first be treated if the glaucoma is to be controlled.

The final stage of any type of uncontrolled glaucoma is blindness. Doctors call this *absolute* glaucoma. The best form of prevention is an annual eye exam.

According to estimates by the National Society for the Prevention of Blindness, nearly two million Americans age thirty-five or over, or one in every fifty of that age group, have glaucoma. Nearly 300,000 new cases occur each year. The Society estimates that one million have the disease but don't know they have it. In 1978, the Society mounted a nationwide glaucoma detection program with the help of their affiliates throughout the country. Since the start of this detection program, hundreds of thousands of men, women and children have taken glaucoma tests. The policy of the Society is to go out into communities to reach as broad a segment of the public as possible. In Georgia, mobile "vision vans" travel from one site to another and set up their testing units on the streets.

The American Academy of Ophthalmology ranks chronic open-angle glaucoma as one of the three leading causes of blindness among all United States inhabitants, but among blacks it ranks number one. The rate of blindness from glaucoma among blacks in the 45-to-65 age group is 14 to 17 times that among whites. Though unable to explain this discrepancy with any certainty, Academy spokesmen suggest that contributing factors are a higher prevalence of abnormal eye pressure early in life, less access to and use of health resources, resulting in a lower rate of early detection and treatment, and poorer compliance in the rigorous treatment. This last is not surprising, considering the economic problems that affect the ability of many blacks to pay for the daily medications that must be taken throughout the lifetime of glaucoma victims.

The Academy alerted its members and other health professionals to the gravity of the glaucoma problem among blacks and the need for widespread screening programs. It recommended that treatment and follow-up of glaucoma in blacks be pursued more aggressively while being "sensitive and attentive to economic and other factors that may interfere with compliance."

In Washington, D.C., where the population is 75 percent black and the blindness rate the highest of any city in the country, the challenge is first to educate this high-risk group about the disastrous course of untreated glaucoma, and second, to develop ways of facilitating eye examinations and treatment. It does little good to tell people in severe economic straits that they have a sight-threatening chronic eye disorder unless there is some provision for financing long-term treatment. Otherwise the problem will remain merely a deplorable statistic.

Besides those four major eye disorders, two other serious impairments must be noted: corneal disorders and retinitis pigmentosa.

Corneal Disorders

Every year in the United States two million cases of corneal disorders are reported, plus 1.7 million cases of injuries requiring medical attention, and it is likely that many more injuries are never reported. Some 62 percent of all acute and chronic afflictions of the eyes involve corneas. Because of its exposed position on the exterior of the eye—the cornea is a transparent cover

over the iris and the pupil—the cornea is vulnerable to scratches, particles that sometimes become embedded in the tissue, and wounds from all manner of sharp edges—knives, broken glass, slivers of metal, toys, tree branches, and cats' claws. If the cornea is damaged, the passage of light is obstructed or distorted, and the retina does not get a clear image.

The cornea is one of the body's most sensitive areas. Pain can be so intense that when a particle hits the cornea our imagination magnifies the size of the particle as if to make it commensurate with the degree of the pain.

In this chemical era, eyes suffer from mild irritations, from smog or noxious emissions from industrial plants, but more serious is eye damage from chemical explosions. The frightful disaster in Bhopal, India, in December 1984 killed from 2,000 to 5,000 (depending on the source of the figures) and injured almost 200,000. Thousands were blinded by ulcers that formed on their corneas.

Ocular herpes (herpes simplex virus) is the leading cause of corneal blindness and visual impairment. Though now treatable with medication, ocular herpes is almost impossible to cure, because the virus becomes latent and may flare up at any time. Of the 500,000 new cases occurring annually, some 50 percent recur. This destructive and capricious virus is the object of intensive research by basic and clinical investigators throughout the Western world.

The cornea is more than a passive conduit for light

into the interior of the eyes. It bends (refracts) light beams entering the eye so they focus properly on the retina, not too far in front or behind it. If the beam focuses too far in front, a person has trouble seeing objects far away, a disorder called *myopia,* or nearsightedness. Most cases of myopia can be corrected with prescription glasses or contact lenses, but degenerative myopia, often present at birth, is a much more serious disorder and can contribute to cataracts, retinal detachment and glaucoma. If the cornea focuses the light beam behind the retina, a person is farsighted, sees well objects at a distance, but not those close up, a condition known as *hyperopia.*

Nearly 100 million Americans have some type of refraction error, either nearsightedness, farsightedness or astigmatism, distorted vision commonly caused by a defect in the curvature of the cornea. In most instances, errors in refraction can be corrected by glasses or contact lenses.

The most dramatic advance in corneal treatment is corneal transplantation, one of the great medical success stories of the twentieth century. In the early part of the century, there were a few tentative attempts at corneal transplantation. The technique has been improved and refined in recent decades.

Today corneal transplantations are the most successful transplant operations being performed, according to Dr. G. Stephen Foster, assistant clinical scientist at the Eye Research Institute of Retina Foundation, in Boston. More than 90 percent of all donor corneas are readily accepted by the eyes that receive them. Success in corneal transplants begins with an evaluation of the corneal disorder and the general health of the eye itself. Patients whose corneas have been burned by chemicals, or who have poorly controlled glaucoma, or an active infection of the eye have no more than a 25 percent chance of a successful transplant. But as in any type of surgery, many factors influence success, and surgeons take these factors into account when deciding whether to operate. Much of the success of corneal transplantation is due to refined surgical techniques, including the use of high-powered surgical microscopes, miniature surgical instruments, "inert" sutures that reduce the possibility of infection, and methods of postoperative care.

Also contributing to the success of corneal transplants is the selection of donor tissue. In the early days of corneal transplants, some fatal diseases, including rabies, were inadvertently transmitted to the recipients of implants. To avoid such complications, tissue donations nowadays are carefully screened and are not used if the donors at the time of death had neurological diseases, cancer, or severe infections. The New York Eye-Bank for Sight Restoration, however, emphasizes that all eyes donated, even though not used for corneal transplants, are invaluable for research on eye disorders.

The National Eye Institute in its five-year plan for vision research spanning the period 1983 to 1987, gives major emphasis to corneal diseases—infections such as herpes simplex virus, disorders of the surface of the eyes, eye medications, contact lenses, refractive errors, congenital disorders, corneal transplantations, and corneal dysfunctions. While its own staff of scientists investigate many of these problems, the Institute's major function is to support vision research in medical centers throughout the country.

Retinitis Pigmentosa

In the 1970s Bill Berger, a successful New York literary agent then in his forties, began having trouble seeing at night. He had first been told he had retinitis pigmentosa in the 1950s, when he was in the Navy. An eye doctor had made the diagnosis in the course of a routine examination; the term meant nothing to Bill at the time, and he paid it no heed. After all, he could see perfectly. When he was well established as an authors' agent, heading his own firm, Berger Associates, he learned that he was going blind. A blind literary agent! Retinitis pigmentosa suddenly was a term fraught with terrifying significance.

He was my agent at the time, but he kept his dread secret and I had no inkling, until I interviewed him for this book, of his desperate search for some treatment that would halt the progress of the disease and enable him to see and to carry on his sight-oriented career.

"I went from one ophthalmologist to another," he told me, recalling that harrowing period.

I tried every aid on the market that might help, and for a while some did help, magnifiers and special lamps. I took mobility training for getting around New York. I had to keep up my contacts with editors and most of that is done at the lunch table. For a long time I wouldn't admit that my sight was failing. I developed all sorts of ruses to cover up. When I was having lunch with editors, I'd pick a restaurant I was familiar with, where I knew the layout. And I always requested a table by the window.

But after a while I knew I wasn't fooling anyone but myself. For a while I had manuscripts read to me by someone on my staff, but that was an expensive use of people whose skills were more important to my business in other ways. Then, through the American Association for the Blind in New York, I learned about the Kurzweil talking machine that reads typed and printed pages. I'm now using a fourth-generation model of that machine. It does my reading for me.

His most important aid, however, is his memory, which he cultivates assiduously. When discussing a manuscript with an editor, he can't read from the manuscript, so he has to remember characters, scenes, plots of novels, and in nonfiction, he has to have at his fingertips the key elements of the subjects and angles that are important for marketing the book.

When I interviewed him, Bill still had minimal residual vision, but it had the disconcerting habit of fluctuating during the day.

When I get up in the morning, my sight is at its best, not very good, but best. As the day goes on, I find that fatigue or stress affects acuity. Weather, too. I see better on rainy days, not foggy, damp days, but rainy days. Why, I don't know. I'm fearful of being out in darkness, and in winter as soon as daylight begins to fade, I cut loose from the office and walk the fourteen blocks to my apartment. I carry a folding white cane now, not so much to guide me as to alert others, especially drivers that I can't see them. Now, I never go out at night unless someone is with me.

Retinitis pigmentosa is one of those visual disorders attributable to bad luck of the genes. It is inherited and incurable, though discoveries by genetic scientists

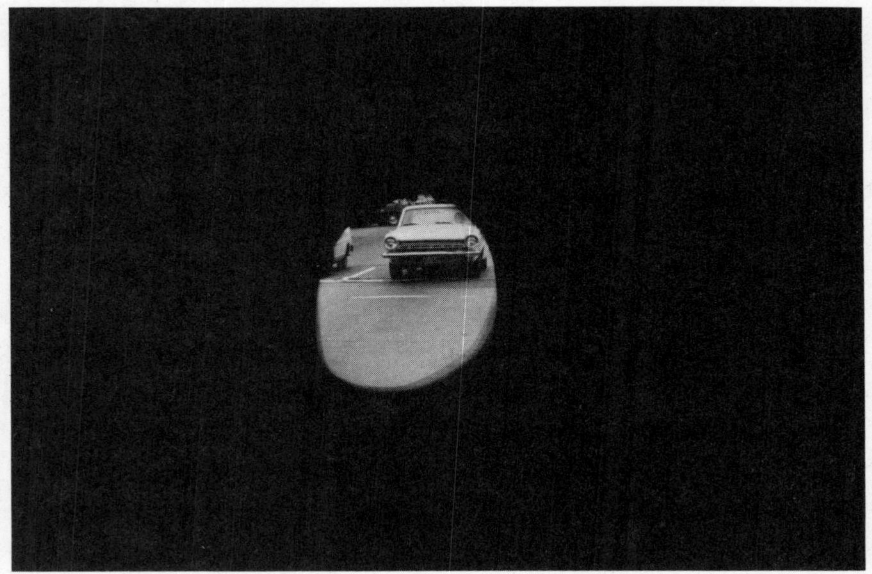

Retinitis Pigmentosa: An inherited disease which affects vision due to a breakdown of retinal tissues. Characterized by night blindness, retinitis pigmentosa frequently results in tunnel vision. Central vision can also be affected. (AMERICAN FOUNDATION FOR THE BLIND)

could obsolete its incurable status. The disease itself results from defective genes that cause the cells of the retina to deteriorate. For a long time it was believed that only males got the disease and that females escaped, but passed on the defective gene to their sons.

Scientists have identified three genetic types of retinitis pigmentosa, each with its special mode of inheritance. The most severe form is X-chromosome-linked, or "sex-linked," accounting for some 30 percent of all cases, an estimated 50,000 to 100,000 in the United States. Even though they have normal vision themselves, one person in fifty carries the defective genes, which impartially afflict all social, ethnic and racial groups. Males, who have only one X chromosome, may suffer such severe retinal damage as to become blind by the time they reach forty years of age. With the protection of their extra X chromosome, females who carry the retinitis pigmentosa gene have milder forms of the disease, if they have it at all. As is true of sex-linked disorders, women can pass on the terrible legacy of blindness to their sons. Today, it's possible for a woman early in pregnancy to find out whether the defective gene is present in the fetus and make a choice about having the baby. Because of three types of retinitis pigmentosa and their modes of inheritance, women diagnosed as carriers can seek genetic counseling, offered by most low vision clinics.

Generally, the first symptom of retinitis pigmentosa in children and in adolescents is difficulty in seeing at night, a difficulty that slowly worsens. Peripheral vision decreases as if a dragnet were slowly being drawn across the retina constricting its field of vision until there may be only a small opening through which a person can see, much like looking through a tunnel to the opening at the far end. In fact, the term *tunnel vision* is commonly used to describe the type of vision characteristic of retinitis pigmentosa. Blindness is not inevitable; many people retain small, but usable "islands of sight" in the retina.

During the slow decline of vision in retinitis pigmentosa numerous low vision aids can be used to enhance remaining sight. Low vision clinics are the best source for these special aids.

Retinitis pigmentosa is not so prevalent as macular degeneration, cataracts, diabetic retinopathy and glaucoma, but its predictable, irreversible course places it among the calamitous eye diseases. Although there is as yet no cure or scientifically proved treatment for it, what augurs well for its eventual control is its clear-cut genetic origin. Geneticists have identified the gene, but so far have not found its location on the chromosomes. Once they make that discovery, retinitis pigmentosa will be a prime target for genetic engineering.

Those who suffer from any type of severe visual impairment or are afraid of becoming victims of disorders that will rob them of their sight should take heart. The good news is that what could not be done to correct some visual defects ten years ago can be done today, and many things that cannot yet be done will most likely become successful in the coming decade.

In the next chapter, we'll visit several low vision clinics and observe at first hand how eye specialists and their staffs are helping patients put their defective vision to maximum use.

4
Low Vision Services

Dr. Eleanor E. Faye, ophthalmological director of the New York Lighthouse Low Vision Services, summarizes the elements of comprehensive low vision services in this way: First, there is the diagnosis of any eye disease, advice on preventing further deterioration and, when indicated, referrals for surgical or other medical correction. Second, optical services beginning with any necessary refraction correction and followed by advice on optical and nonoptical aids for enhancing residual vision. And third, instruction in the use of the aids and psychosocial and rehabilitation services. "It is attention to these special needs," Dr. Faye says in her book, *Clinical Low Vision,*

> that sets low vision services apart from routine eye care. As low vision is recognized by professional eye-care doc-

> tors, the public, and legislators as an entity distinctly different from blindness, low vision services will expand to the benefit of millions of partially sighted men, women, and children. A doctor cannot say "Nothing more can be done" when there is a large body of knowledge to the contrary.

In the late 1950s there were about five low vision clinics in the United States. Thirty years later there are hundreds, not only in this country, but also in Canada, England, and other western European countries. In the span of those three decades, the concept of the best use of residual vision has attracted hundreds of eye-care doctors and therapists and thousands of patients, as word spreads about the new specialty that keeps the partially sighted out of the blindness system.

At the outset, there were no guidelines for setting up low vision clinics or standards for staffing them. The clinics developed independently, their characteristics determined by their directors and in some instances by the schools and institutions housing them. Though many of the clinics are directed by ophthalmologists, most are under the direction of optometrists.

The distinction between these two professions is not clear-cut in the minds of most people. One reason for this confusion is that in several areas, the functions of these two types of eye-care specialists overlap, particularly in regard to eye examinations. This overlap not only accounts for some of the confusion, but unfortunately, causes considerable friction between the two professions. Because it is important in their own self-interest that patients understand the roles of the ophthalmologist and optometrist in treatment programs, here are definitions that should help clarify those roles:

An *ophthalmologist* is a medical doctor (M.D.) who has completed four years of medical school and goes on to four or more years of training in diagnosing and treating eye diseases and defects with medication or surgery. Ophthalmologists also test vision acuity and prescribe corrective lenses. Advances in diagnostic and surgical techniques (corneal transplants, cataract removal and lens implants, retinal repair, and most recently vitrectomy) have attracted an increasing number of ophthalmological doctors into what have become important and lucrative subspecialties. Ophthalmologists were pioneers in promoting the low vision concept and many of them specialize in low vision services.

An *optometrist* holds the degree of doctor of optometry (O.D.), awarded after completion of the four-year professional optometry course. Low vision care is now required training for the O.D. degree and for certification to practice optometry. Their training emphasizes the diagnosis of vision problems and assessing the health and efficiency of the eyes, not only the near and distant acuities but, in their low vision work, how adequately the eyes function in everyday situations. When there is evidence of disease in the eyes or corrective surgery is indicated, optometrists refer patients to opthalmologists or other physicians. Optometrists prescribe corrective spectacles and contact lenses and, for partially sighted patients, low vision aids.

It is the *optician* who dispenses glasses and contact

lenses (usually corrective) and low vision aids prescribed by eye doctors.

Low vision services is a term that encompasses a great diversity of facilities, staffs and services. Clinics range from a one-person operation (sometimes a technician rather than an eye doctor) with services limited to eye examinations and prescription of aids, to large, well-organized clinics staffed by multidisciplinary teams of eye doctors, specialists in low vision assessment and in the selection of aids and training in their use, social workers, psychologists, coordinators of patient services, and counselors of patients and their families. Whatever the nature of these clinics, all share the one goal: to help patients use their remaining vision with maximum efficiency.

"Every week, at least one patient being admitted to our low vision clinic says that an eye doctor has told them they're going blind and that nothing can be done for them," Robert Cope, counselor at the William Feinbloom Vision Rehabilitation Center at the Pennsylvania College of Optometry, in Philadelphia, told me in an interview.

> What many of these doctors are saying is, "If I can't help you, no one can."
>
> There's a strong element of professional ego involved in that attitude. It's hard for some established eye doctors even to admit that another professional could do what they can't do for a patient or to admit there's a new type of eye-care service they don't know much about. Either way, not being able to help a patient can make a doctor very defensive.

Cutting patients adrift without hope is such a devastating experience that some patients, suddenly told they were going blind and that nothing could be done for them, have committed suicide. Others have given up jobs, and in a sense have become blind, years before completely losing their sight; though eye doctors can predict eventual blindness, they may never know exactly when this will happen. Some patients with declining vision have functioned for years before losing their eyesight.

Before taking a look at several clinics, let's consider another source of low vision services: private practitioners specializing in these services. This is a type of practice few eye doctors can afford on a full-time basis. Compared to a routine eye examination, the low vision examination is complex and time consuming, requiring at least one hour, usually longer, and sometimes several sessions spread out over weeks if vision fluctuates or if the patient is elderly and easily fatigued by the examination.

The vision assessment includes an examination of the interior of the eyes, tests of near, distant and peripheral vision, eye and eye-muscle coordination, refraction, and color vision, this last to determine possible damage to the macula and optic nerves. Then comes the selection of low vision aids. Sometimes one aid suffices for a particular task of primary importance to a patient, but two or more aids may be necessary for different tasks at different distances. The patient must be trained in using the aids; in certain types of visual problem, such as macular degeneration and the loss of "straight-ahead" vision, patients are taught to see eccentrically—that is, to use other parts of the retina in place of the macula.

As a young practitioner describes this type of service,

> Low vision is a new frontier in eye care and I like being part of it and influencing its development. And it's inherently an optimistic type of service. In most cases, you can do something to help these people and it's a very exciting and gratifying thing. It's not a routine, assembly-line type of practice. You're dealing not only with the eyes, but with the whole person, including the patient's lifestyle and with fears and frustrations that go along with seriously defective, but usable vision.

Most partially sighted people who come to low vision clinics have traveled a discouraging route through the offices of many eye doctors, have failed many eye examinations, and are haunted by the specter of *blindness,* a word seldom explained to them. (How blind or in what way blind?) Understandably they are apprehensive about yet another doctor and more eye examinations. Some bring with them not only fear and hopelessness, but, as if that were not burden enough, add to it a sense of guilt, attributing their eye problems to punishment for some wrongdoing.

Uppermost in the minds of most patients dismissed by eye doctors as being beyond help is their fear of going blind. "Blindness is grossly misunderstood," said Counselor Robert Cope, who, legally blind himself from retinitis pigmentosa, interviews new patients with empathy based on his own experience.

Most people think absence of light is something insupportable, but they should understand that vision is a mental activity, the mental component of a learned activity. The brain interprets what the eyes see. It's possible to live without vision. Loss of sight is something that happens. One's priorities shift. The important thing, as I tell patients, is to keep doing what one has to do, to keep active, to be flexible in making changes and, when necessary, to adapt.

Vision can slowly deteriorate over five to eighteen, even more, years without a patient's needing optical aids. This is especially true in some cases of macular degeneration [Mr. Cope said]. These days many congenital eye disabilities can be corrected. Some patients born blind, through corrective surgery or a custom-designed optical aid may be in their twenties or thirties, even older, when they see for the first time.

People must decide what they want to see. To say "I want to see better" is too general and of little help to an eye-care specialist, who at some point must select aids appropriate for what the patient wants to see.

Patients who are reluctantly brought to the Center by their grown-up children or other relatives are not likely to succeed in the treatment program.

A seventy-year-old retired man was brought here by his son and daughter. He could no longer see to read, but his great pleasure was being read to by his children. It was not just the reading itself that meant so much to him, but their company. It satisfied an inner need for their presence and his dependence on them. Needless to say, he resisted any aids that would have enabled him to do his own reading. This is not an unusual situation—lonely, elderly parents clinging to children, unaware in many instances of the burden they put on young parents who have jobs and their own children to manage.

They reject anything that would enhance their vision and make them less dependent. Some aids are strange-looking—telescopic lenses, for instance—and require practice and skill in their use, which many elderly patients aren't willing to work at. Sometimes, of course, their physical condition makes such effort too difficult. We try to identify these people before they get into the treatment system, for they prevent highly motivated patients from benefiting from services that are in great demand. But we're careful about making snap judgments. You can't always tell what inner resources and determination some elderly people have. There can be some real surprises.

The Feinbloom Center schedules a series of three appointments for each patient. Before the first appointment, the clinic sends the patient an information packet explaining low vision services, potential benefits of optical aids, and a preview of what will take place on each clinic visit. (These visits are scheduled three weeks apart.)

The first visit is a half-hour "intake" session (a medical and social history, as described earlier), followed by an assessment of visual acuities, refraction, visual fields, binocularity, and a comprehensive eye-health evaluation, all this taking about one to two or more hours. On the second visit, eye-care specialists help patients select optical or nonoptical aids for specific tasks and instruct patients in their use. Generally the

Center lends aids for patients to try out at home, the work place or school, and in getting about. On the third visit, the effectiveness of the loaned aids is evaluated and those decided on are ordered. When necessary, patients are given additional instructions in their use.

That formal schedule has built-in flexibility, Dr. Richard L. Brilliant, the Center director, explains:

> Patients may have concerns, fears, and hesitations about undertaking their rehabilitation program, so we arrange for members of the social service staff to meet with them and give them a chance to talk about those concerns. Sometimes it's helpful for patients to bring along a member of the family to this meeting; support of the family is essential. Occasionally, patients want a husband or wife to be present at the eye examination and during the selection of aids, something we certainly allow. Sometimes during an initial visual assessment, we realize that a patient, for various reasons, sometimes psychological, may not be a good candidate for low vision services. We discuss the situation with them and, if they decide to drop out, we feel that at least they have had a thorough refraction and ocular assessment.

One purpose in separating the visits, according to Dr. Brilliant, is that on the first visit patients are shown sample optical aids to prepare them for the physical appearance of some of the bizarre-looking aids. By separating the rigorous visual-assessment session from the selection of optical aids, patients are more alert and receptive to training in their use. As part of patient education, each supervising doctor summarizes the findings of the examination and gives a copy of the report to the patient, as well as to the referring physician.

The "patient's advocate," usually an optometric intern, keeps in touch with the patient throughout the entire rehabilitation process, developing a personal rapport that makes it easier for patients to talk more freely about their reactions. If there are transportation difficulties, the social service staff calls on community agencies for help. A certain number of patients who are unable to pay the fees are subsidized through various means, but the clinic is largely supported by patient fees.

When the Center opened, in 1978, only eight of 150 students in the Pennsylvania College of Optometry applied for low vision training. In 1985, forty interns were accepted from seventy-five who applied. "This reflects the increased interest in low vision among optometrists and I think there's also the fact that the clinic is attractive and the atmosphere, though high-pressured, is casual. It takes a lot of strenuous effort to maintain that casual atmosphere," Dr. Brilliant said with a little smile. "The intern program is very important, for when these interns go into practice as optometrists, they will know what can be done for patients with partial sight. We're instilling in these young people not only an understanding of low vision, but a commitment to this type of service."

Though careful screening of applicants for services

accounts to some extent for the 85 to 95 percent success rate in helping patients use their residual vision, the primary factor in this success is patient motivation. The stronger a patient's desire to improve vision for whatever reasons, the greater the likelihood of achieving that goal. A happy surprise for many patients—and for the eye doctors as well—is the discovery during the eye examination that the patient has far more usable vision than he or she realized. It's not unusual for patients who can't read newsprint or the largest letters on an eye chart twenty feet away to think they are blind. The problem may be one of poor refraction, a defect that usually can be corrected by prescription glasses or contact lenses. Some agitated patients, fearful that their failing vision means that they are going blind, are ecstatic when the eye examiner tells them that all they need to increase their visual acuity is a simple magnifying glass.

A patient who won the hearts of the Center staff was a workman from a small village in Yugoslavia who had in some way heard about the Center and, though almost blind and speaking no English, made his way to Philadelphia, his fare paid by money raised by neighbors in his village. He found not only the clinic but a Yugoslavian priest, who, through a local radio station, appealed to the Yugoslavian community in Philadelphia for help. The radio station was inundated with offers of help, invitations to stay with families while he was being treated at the clinic, and even an invitation to share Thanksgiving dinner.

Dr. Charles F. Mullen, executive director of the Eye Institute, of which the Center is a component, added the happy ending. "We gave him an optical device that enabled him to return to Yugoslavia and go back to work. Since then we've had many patients from Yugoslavia who heard about his experience."

The visual assessment is the reference point for all low vision services. When the assessment indicates that surgical or other medical treatment is appropriate, patients are advised to have that treatment before going on with the low vision treatment. The length of time the assessment takes varies from clinic to clinic and from patient to patient. Dr. Randall T. Jose, an optometrist, coordinator of rehabilitative optometry at the University of Houston's College of Optometry and editor of the book *Understanding Low Vision,* favors an assessment of from eight to ten hours, spaced over several sessions. The low vision clinic he formerly directed and now oversees as a part of a broader vision rehabilitation program, has on its staff eye doctors, instructors in the use of visual aids and in eccentric viewing, a social worker, a psychologist, and a mobility trainer. The tone of the clinic is expressed in the style of clothes worn by the staff. Dr. Jose believes the "white coat" can be disconcerting to many patients, especially to those who have spent a lot of time in hospitals and clinics. So, in examination rooms and corridors staff members are dressed in sports clothes and handsome Texas boots.

About seventy patients are admitted to the clinic

each year, their ages ranging from nine months to ninety years and over. Macular degeneration, the most common eye defect seen at the clinic, is treated with special aids and training in eccentric viewing, the technique that uses retinal cells outside the macula to compensate for the loss of central vision. Because most visual defects occur in the elderly, the clinic is affiliated with the geriatric unit of the University of Houston's College of Optometry.

Dr. Jose believes that the patients most likely to benefit from low vision services are those with specific visual objectives.

> Just to say "I want to see better" doesn't help us get at the problem. The patient must identify specific objectives, whether it's to get from home to work, to cook, to read, or watch ball games. But we find that patients often tell us one thing, when what they really want is to have their former good vision restored. We try to bring them around to accepting more realistic goals.
>
> Quite a few of our patients are business executives who come to us because they refuse to be lumped in with the blind. They usually don't know much about low vision services, but they do know they need help, and they think we may be able to give it to them. As executives they are embarrassed by their failing vision and their inability to see to read, for in a sense they've become illiterates. Because they're strongly motivated and intelligent, they're excellent patients to work with.

The patient's routine begins with a preassessment interview with a social worker, who goes into the nature of the visual disability, how it affects the patient's life, living patterns at home, work or school, and its effects on family and social relationships. The patient also is asked about travel problems, whether he or she gets about freely or is confined to the house. In this interview, the patient's objectives are discussed. This preassessment sometimes reveals that the patient doesn't want low vision services, but has been coerced, by family or business associates, into going to the clinic. There are no rules for handling this situation, but one thing is for sure, there is no coercion on the part of the clinic staff.

Besides referrals from doctors and teachers, many come from the Texas State Commission for the Blind, which, according to Dr. Jose, is one of the most progressive in the country, giving a high priority to vision. The Commission reimburses the clinic for part of the cost of some services.

When a patient is accepted, the next step is the eye examination, which tells the doctor and the patient what they have to work with, the stability of any disease process, the amount of intact retina that is left, and the quality of the visual receptor cells in the retina. If it is decided at that point that surgical procedures or other medical treatment could substantially improve the patient's vision, the patient is referred to an ophthalmologist.

> Our services are complementary to those of the ophthalmologists, who consider them a resource rather than

competition [Dr. Jose says]. After we are assured that all medical and surgical treatment has been provided, we assess peripheral and central fields of vision. This information is essential not only for prescribing optical and other aids, but for use by mobility instructors in evaluating a patient's functional vision. Before considering magnification aids, the examiner tests for possible refraction problems. We don't take it for granted that everyone goes to eye doctors. Some patients who come to the clinic get an eye examination for the first time in their lives.

More than 60 percent of the partially sighted population suffers unnecessary visual impairment because of poor refraction, which usually can be corrected by prescription lenses. "We do a thorough examination of the optical components of the patients' visual systems to make sure the loss of acuity is due to pathology and not to a poor refraction," says Dr. Jose. "We measure acuity at both distance and near, not only as a basis for selecting optical aids, but also as a useful base for judging a patient's ability to function in nonclinical settings."

The next stage is the selection of optical aids appropriate for whatever tasks the patient has specified. Some unique tasks call for specially designed aids. An insurance salesman requested an aid that would bring the faces of his clients into sharp focus. The optical designer at the clinic implanted a prism that looked like a small pale-blue lozenge into a lens of the salesman's half-glasses. At the clinic I tried on this device and was astonished to see that faces, suddenly enlarged, came at me like movie close-ups. With that device, the salesman would have no difficulty seeing his clients' faces in sharp detail.

Patients are allowed to borrow aids for a trial period. When they return to the clinic, they report on the effectiveness of the aids. Sometimes adjustments are necessary, and sometimes a different aid is selected or additional aids for specific seeing tasks. When feasible, a member of the clinic staff visits patients in their customary settings, at home, work place, or school, to assess how effective the aids are outside the clinic, which is a structured setting that in itself enhances the ability to see well. Outside, other factors like lighting, arrangement of desks, noise from machinery or from other people, influence how well a person sees. This kind of realistic assessment may lead to changes in aids or to the prescription of additional aids for certain tasks or settings.

During the course of the treatment program, social workers, mobility instructors, and in some instances, the psychologist contribute their observations to the patient's evaluation. The clinicians in turn report their findings to members of the rehabilitation team, thus ensuring the best possible solution for the patient's visual and related problems. While the patients are the focus of this communications network, they are also an integral part of it. They are urged to express their feelings about what is going on, their reactions to the examination, aids and training. Some patients say the most important part of the treatment program is the eye examination itself. Others pick out the training in the use of the aids, still others the mobility training. Some patients give top rating to the services provided by the social workers. The emphasis changes with each patient. "Or, at least it should," says Dr. Jose. "If it doesn't, something is wrong with the system. It's not getting at individual needs. They're different with each patient."

Dr. Jose extends the low vision work of the clinic through the *Journal of Vision Rehabilitation,* which he founded and edits. Primarily for professionals, the *Journal* covers all aspects of low vision and keeps readers up-to-date with developments in training, new types of aids, computers, and such controversial topics as driving permits for the partially sighted.

A low vision clinic that treats patients who have a disease-related visual problem is in the W. P. Beetham Eye Clinic of the Joslin Diabetes Foundation, in Boston. Diabetes accounts for thousands of new cases of blindness each year. Before the discovery of insulin, few people survived diabetes, but today with the high survival rate, impaired vision is one of the unfortunate consequences of the disease. Diabetes causes a proliferation of blood vessels in the eyes and, unless controlled in the early stages, can lead to blindness. Known as *diabetic retinopathy,* this blinding eye disease takes a slow, progressive course.

Director of the low vision clinic, Dr. Richard M. Calderon, an optometrist, told me that patients in most low vision clinics are generally in good health except for their eye problems. "But in this clinic, we are dealing with people who have a chronic, incurable disease. The threat of total vision loss adds to their anxieties and is one that eye doctors must handle with great understanding and tact."

When patients come to the low vision clinic, Dr. Calderon looks for certain clues about them; even before beginning the interview. "I observe, for instance, how the person walks, whether the gait is confident and assured or shuffling and uncertain, the person's posture and manner. These observations give me some idea of the person I'll be dealing with."

In the first interview, Dr. Calderon asks the patient about the nature of the eye problem and when it first manifested itself. "I ask them about themselves, who they are, what they do, and what they want and expect to do. Together, the patient and I make a list of those wants and expectations and discuss each item on the list. There may be a difference between what seems important to me as the eye doctor and what seems most important to the patient. We work out these differences and then set goals that can be achieved fairly quickly, whether it's corrective surgical or other medical treatment. I explain the nature of the eye problem and outline the treatment program."

During the first interview, Dr. Calderon emphasized, an eye doctor must keep in mind that the patient is tense and apprehensive. "The patient's internal noise level may be so high he or she does not hear what the doctor is saying. It may be necessary at a subsequent visit to go over everything again when that inner noise level is greatly reduced and fears allayed. Sometimes, I even have to reintroduce myself to patients."

After the vision assessment, depending on the patient's eye condition and goals, Dr. Calderon prescribes one or more aids and instructs the patient in their use. Of great concern to patients taking insulin is being able to see to load a syringe. For those patients, there are special aids that enable them to do that.

From the beginning of his low vision treatment program, Dr. Calderon counsels patients on coping with declining vision. Though his clinic is a one-man operation, he draws on the expertise of the multidisciplinary staff of the W.P. Beetham Eye Clinic for consultation and services, including surgical and medical treatment.

> We prepare patients for those disturbing fluctuations in visual acuity related to blood sugar levels. If the blood sugar is up, patients become more nearsighted. Our lens prescriptions must be related to these changes in blood sugar levels. In this clinic, we cannot separate the eye problem from the systemic problem of diabetes. Some patients simply cannot believe what doctors tell them about their condition and how important it is to follow instructions about diet, drinking and smoking. What we strive to get over to them is that the risk of visual impairment ties in directly with the control of their disease. It requires a delicate balance between scaring a patient into a nothing-can-help-me frame of mind and a to-hell-with-it attitude. We try to get them to accept the fact that, indeed, they can do a great deal for their own health and vision. In all

this we also try to increase a patient's appreciation of his or her eyes as vital tools of existence.

Diabetics, Dr. Calderon says, need continuing eye-care services, checkups on the eyes to detect incipient problems and for control of existing conditions.

Diabetics who prefer contact lenses sometimes have difficulty in getting a proper evaluation of the status of their eyes. Unless the eye examiner understands how diabetes affects the eyes, problems may go undetected, a situation that could result in irrevocable sight loss. Contact lenses for diabetics present special problems because they must be properly prescribed to compensate for some of the eye defects caused by the disease.

The most common eye problems encountered at the Beetham Eye Clinic are diabetic retinopathy, cataracts, glaucoma, including neurovascular glaucoma related to diabetes, and macular degeneration, which is apt to occur earlier in diabetics than in the rest of the population.

It was not until 1981 that low vision service standards were established by a special commission under the aegis of the National Accreditation Council of Agencies Serving the Blind and Handicapped. But even before those standards were formally established, many low vision clinics were already operating according to similar principles.

One such clinic is the Pacific Medical Center Low Vision Services in San Francisco, affiliated with Presbyterian Hospital and the San Francisco Lighthouse. A multidisciplinary clinic, it admits some 570 new patients a year and averages three patients four mornings a week. The age range of patients is from infants to a few in their nineties, and an occasional patient over one hundred years old.

Clinic director Dr. August Colenbrander, an ophthalmologist born in the Netherlands, began his education in visual problems early, when as a boy he accompanied his father, head of Leiden (then Leyden) School of Ophthalmology, on tours of institutions for the blind. Then Queen Juliana, whose daughter Christina was born with severely impaired vision, through her personal interest in the visual problems of children put the Netherlands in the forefront of systems of care for visually impaired children.

Dr. Colenbrander puts great store on properly defining visual problems. "More people are blinded by definition than by any other cause," he says. Dr. Colenbrander, as you may recall from a previous chapter, was instrumental in the codification of low vision as a special category in the 1979 edition of WHO's International Classification of Diseases.

His own set of definitions for visual problems consists of four categories: disorder (anatomical), impairment (functional); disability (how a person functions), and handicap (the person related to the social setting). "Low vision patients need help in all four areas," he told me in an interview. "A wheelchair reduces a handicap by changing the environment, but it does not reduce the disability. One way to reduce the handicap of partial sight, for instance, is to live in a house where everything is on one floor, a ranch-style house rather than one with flights of stairs."

In the clinic that he directs, Dr. Colenbrander and other eye-care specialists deal with the "disorder" and "impairment" aspects of partial sight. A coordinator for patient services handles the disability and handicap aspects, including referring patients to community agencies such as the San Francisco Lighthouse for visual rehabilitation services.

A major part of the clinic's activities is a training program for ophthalmology hospital residents that emphasizes low vision services as part of modern eye-care service. Some residents return at the end of their residency for refresher training in low vision. As one resident put it, "Things are changing so rapidly—new optical and nonoptical aids, new techniques of training in their use, and new rehabilitation methods—that even those of us working every day in the low vision field have difficulty keeping up with developments."

According to Dr. Colenbrander, many ophthalmologists and optometrists don't know about the wide choice of aids. "Some are not inclined to learn. They're satisfied to continue giving traditional acuity tests, though such tests do not evaluate a patient's functional capacity. Low vision assessments take much more time than the usual acuity tests and cut into the doctor's productivity. But as more doctors learn about low vision services, they are more inclined to refer patients."

Youngsters between six and twenty years of age are the most difficult patients to deal with, Dr. Colenbrander says. "They resist wearing bizarre-looking aids, and our clinic staff has to call on parents and teachers to encourage these youngsters to use them. Teachers especially can do a great deal to enlist the support of classmates of partially sighted students by explaining the importance of those optical aids to the student's advancement in learning. Peer rejection is, unfortunately, a factor in the bland, give-up attitude of so many young, near-blind students."

The clinic staff talk proudly about their successes, one a one-hundred-one-year-old man who lives alone, does his own cooking, takes care of his house, and indulges in his favorite pastime, reading. Running close second to that man in staff esteem is the eighty-seven-year-old businessman who wears a pair of specially designed half-glasses with an inserted prism for magnification and manages his own business as a manufacturer's representative.

Many patients have a "cure-on-demand" attitude toward physicians—that is, they expect the doctor to do something that will cure whatever is the matter with them. "Partially sighted patients are apt to come to us with much that same attitude," says Dr. Colenbrander.

To some extent an eye surgeon can comply with that demand by removing cataracts, implanting corneas, or repairing torn retinas. But when it comes to the best use of residual vision, given special aids and training, patients must do that job themselves. No one else can do it for them. I tell patients, "I can show the aids to you, but you must select what is best for you. They must be tailored to your environment. And you must learn to use them." This is not what patients with the "cure-on-demand" attitude like to hear. But I believe patients should work at their own treatment and not leave everything up to the doctor. Low vision treatment is one situation in which patients have considerable control over what will happen to them.

This is just a sampling of low vision clinics. Most of these clinics are multidisciplinary and, in addition to the individualized training given patients, conduct training programs for students in colleges of optometry and for residents in hospital ophthalmology departments. They also provide guidance to eye-care specialists on setting up low vision clinics. At the Keeler Low Vision Clinic in London (one of a network of Keeler low vision clinics throughout England), I met two eye specialists from Yugoslavia who were planning low vision services in that country. Dr. A. William Pratt, director of Vancouver General Hospital Low Vision Clinic, told me that he and his associate had spent a week at Dr. Colenbrander's clinic in San Francisco in preparation for opening their clinic. Directors of low vision clinics welcome observers seeking information about treatment programs and clinic management, a form of "networking" invaluable to the development of low vision services. Most multidisciplinary clinics conduct public-education programs on low vision through printed materials and talks at meetings and on radio and television. The future of low vision services is assured not only by the soundness of the concept, but by the enthusiasm and dedication of the practitioners in this burgeoning specialty.

In the next chapter, we'll discuss some specific ways in which low vision clinics help the partially sighted enhance their usable vision.

5
Low Vision Aids

Taken in the broadest sense, whatever helps the partially sighted to see more clearly and function more efficiently can be considered a low vision aid. In this chapter we'll discuss optical and nonoptical aids.

The optical aids we're most familiar with are eyeglasses and contact lenses, prescription lenses for increasing visual acuity or correcting defects such as near- or far-sightedness. Glasses and contact lenses, widely used as "treatment options" for low vision, are custom tailored to each patient's visual and functional needs following a low vision assessment. But low vision optical aids include an array of special optical devices designed to enhance each patient's usable vision—"islands of sight"—that eye examiners discover during the low vision assessment. These optical devices are classified as "eyewear," though some, like certain types of magnifiers and binoculars, are carried by the partially sighted and used for special viewing tasks.

Nonoptical aids, sometimes called "accessory aids," include large print publications, special dials for telephones and stoves, writing guides and lamps, to name a few. In a special category are the electronic aids, most of them magnifiers, that project onto screens printed and typed materials magnified as much as sixty times the original size. Electronic reading machines and "talking computers" are also eliminating visual barriers to business and academic careers.

Almost every low vision specialist I interviewed cautioned me about giving patients unrealistic expectations about what these aids can do. A common misconception among the partially sighted is that in some miraculous way low vision aids will cure eye defects. Surgery in many instances can correct defects of the lens, cornea, vitreous or retina, but optical aids only enhance usable vision. Nor is an optical aid the best solution of every low vision problem, which can sometimes be solved by adjustments in home or office lighting or the use of color contrast in walls and furniture. Some patients, especially children and young adults who go to low vision clinics and who have never had an eye examination, discover that their poor vision resulted from faulty refraction of the beams of light entering their eyes, a defect correctable by prescription lenses.

Eye-care specialists emphasize that research and technology are constantly coming up with solutions to vision disorders, designing and manufacturing new types of optical and nonoptical aids, and developing new training techniques in the use of aids and in ways the partially sighted can function more efficiently in a sighted world. Even eye-care specialists admit they have a hard time keeping up with developments. But right now there are countless aids for enhancing vision. The trouble is that thousands of people who could benefit from them don't know about them.

Low Vision Assessment

Central to a low vision treatment program is the assessment of the patient's residual vision and determining ways of enhancing it relative to the patient's goals. Unlike a routine eye examination with its subtle confrontational aspect—the doctor looking for defects and the patient apprehensive and defensive—the low vision examiner approaches the assessment from a different point of view. As Dr. Economon puts it, "The low vision examination is a search for abilities, not disabilities."

Though procedures may vary from one clinic to another, within a generally similar framework, low vision assessments include an overview of the patient's general and optical health, family optical history (important for clues to possible hereditary eye defects), marital status, occupation, special interests such as hobbies, sports, and volunteer and community service. An eye doctor then thoroughly examines the exterior and interior of the eye for signs of disease or damage and evaluates the status of the eye condition that is causing low vision, and whether the condition is stable or likely to deteriorate rapidly or gradually over a long period of time as usually occurs with cataracts and macular degeneration.

The acuities tests measure near, intermediate and far vision. Using eye charts developed especially for low vision assessment, the examiner tests the eyes for acuity and for possible refractive errors that must be corrected before optical aids are prescribed. Dr. Economon begins acuity tests using cards with letters as large as ten or more inches high and an inch or so wide. "We bring these cards up to the patients until they can read the letters. Some patients whose sight has deteriorated to the point at which they can no longer read print or distinguish faces are convinced they are blind, but are too chagrined to admit it until some personal crisis forces them to seek help. When these patients discover that they can see those large letters and realize that they are not blind, their relief is overwhelming. It's not unusual for them to weep for joy."

Partially sighted small children and others unable to read letters on charts (foreigners unfamiliar with the Roman alphabet, illiterates, and some mentally retarded children and adults) are given visual-acuity tests using pictures of familiar objects (cars, trees, dogs, etc.) instead of letters. Today electronic diagnostic instruments are used to test the vision of infants, enabling doctors to detect within weeks of birth signs of congenital defects that can be treated surgically or by other medical means.

The acuity test includes an assessment of peripheral vision, the surrounding area you see while looking straight ahead. For many partially sighted people—those, for instance, who have macular degeneration—that area may be the only usable "seeing" area, the visual field that may have to take over some of the functions of defective central vision. There are several ways of assessing field vision. In a test of my field vision, the examiner seated me in front of a large black chart bisected by two white lines joining a white dot in the middle and told me to keep my eyes fixed on the white dot as he moved a pointer through the segments on the chart. Peripherally, my eyes followed the tip of the pointer. If I lost sight of that tip, I said so, and the examiner marked the area on the chart. By the end of the test, he had a map of viable areas of my retina, those "islands of sight" that must be located before a customized aid can be prescribed.

Tests of intermediate vision acuity, as well as near and far vision, are more essential than ever in this age of typewriters and computers. This is why it is important to explain one's occupation—so an eye examiner has a better basis for assessing functional vision and prescribing suitable aids.

In low vision treatment, functional vision is generally considered more important than visual acuity. But assessing functional vision is not quite so straightforward as measuring acuity. Important as it is, most low vision specialists can't even agree on a definition of functional vision. In his book *Management of Low Vision,* Dr. Gerald E. Fonda, one of the first ophthalmologists to advocate low vision services, defines functional vision as "individual vision performance, and consequently, there is no unit of measurement. I define functional vision as the numerical vision (Snellen fraction) modified by intelligence, education, motivation, endurance and experience. For example, an intelligent, highly motivated person with 5/200 vision can often perform better visually than a depressed or retarded person with 20/100 vision." Dr. Fonda goes on to say that it is possible to estimate the degree of functional vision during the diagnostic examination and testing for visual aids and from an appraisal of the patient's educational, vocational and social expectations.

Underscoring the importance it places on assessing functional vision in those with severely impaired sight, the Low Vision Center at Retina Associates in Boston has developed "simulation units" which duplicate different environments—offices, factories, kitchens and classrooms, as well as light conditions in various geographic areas in the world from which patients come to the Center for treatment.

"In these simulated environments," says Dr. Gerald R. Friedman, the Center director,

> we test different types of aids to find out which work best for the patient in a particular setting. For instance, patients from the Middle East with its intense light need

different types of aids from those required for the more subdued light in northern countries. For one of our patients, a lawyer hypersensitive to the bright lights in his office, we simulated that situation and prescribed an aid that enabled him to work comfortably in his office. We find that trying out aids in the simulated environment not only helps in selecting the most effective aids, but cuts down on patients' rejecting them.

In the low vision assessment, examiners consider more than visual aids themselves. The most effective aid for enhancing a patient's residual vision may have to be bypassed if other than visual impairments make it difficult for the patient to use the aid. Patients whose hands are crippled by arthritis or partially paralyzed or tremble uncontrollably will not be able to use certain hand-held aids. Tactful eye doctors or their assistants spare such patients by simply not demonstrating aids they can't cope with, but showing aids the patients can manage, such as stand magnifiers.

We take for granted the rigorous training that ophthalmologists, optometrists, therapists, social workers and special low vision educators have gone through to equip themselves to help patients ameliorate vision problems. Rarely does it occur to patients that they too have some responsibility in this process.

Some medications for treatment of eye disorders or systemic diseases can affect vision. It is important to tell the eye examiner right away about any medication you are taking or have taken in recent months. Unless the examiner knows about your medications, he or she could be misled by drug-caused visual anomalies such as unequal pupil size, color-vision disorders, temporary blindness, double vision and increased sensitivity to light.

Be ready to tell the examiner about how your impaired vision prevents you from doing what you would very much like to do. If the low vision program you are undertaking improves your ability to see, what are some activities you would engage in that you have had to forgo because of poor vision? Would improved vision change any of your long-range goals? Answers to those questions will help the examiner appraise your functional vision.

Take along any visual aids you've been using and items you cannot read easily, items like medicine-bottle labels, Stock Exchange listings, small-print instructions, maps, pages from your daily newspaper, handwritten letters, bank statements, or a Bible. For post-eye-examination comfort, take with you a pair of dark glasses. Coming out into bright sunlight while the pupils of the eyes are still dilated is a painful, tearful, and even blinding experience.

One thing is certain: the more thoroughly you prepare for the low vision assessment, the better it will go. For one thing, your preparation will foster a good rapport between you and the examiner, a factor rarely mentioned in medical publications, but of subtle essentiality to the success of any treatment program. An obvious desire on your part to improve your vision will give the clinic staff one more clue, a very favorable one, about you as a person and as a patient.

Optical Aids

At the rate low vision aids are coming into the market it's difficult even for low vision specialists to keep up with them. Small wonder, then, that so many eye doctors whose practice consists largely of giving traditional eye examinations and prescribing conventional eyewear know so little about the means for enhancing the vision of the partially sighted—not only new types of optical and nonoptical aids, but new methods of retraining the eyes, and innovative techniques for coping with daily living despite visual impairments.

Optical aids have been used for centuries, starting out as hand-held magnifiers, lenses of transparent, polished stones—beryl, quartz and crystal—used by scholars and scribes in monasteries and temples where sacred manuscripts were transcribed, illuminated and studied. Not the needs of scholars but of commerce gave the impetus to optical developments in the nineteenth century. Industry and the great expansion of national and international trade inaugurated the "paper age" that required records of all sorts and clerks who could write and read them. Public education became a commercial necessity. In that dingy, candlelighted era of expanding commerce, the eyes of clerks needed reinforcement, and eyeglasses became widely used.

A revolution in eyewear was the development of contact lenses, based on optical concepts Leonardo da Vinci set forth five hundred years earlier. It took a long time, several decades, for contact lenses to be widely accepted. People were afraid of them and, at first, there were some grounds for public wariness about these magical glass aids that fitted on the eye itself. But plastic contact lenses, less hazardous and easier to take care of, gradually supplanted glass contacts.

While designers of conventional eyewear were concentrating on improving the vision of the average person, no one was paying much attention to the millions of Americans whose sight could not be improved by conventional glasses and contact lenses. Much credit for recognizing the special needs of people with low vision must go to William Feinbloom, the optical genius who recognized the special visual needs of the partially sighted and applied his skills to designing optical aids for them. Many low vision optical aids prescribed today are based on his optical concepts. Throughout his life he continued to design low vision aids. Not long before he died in 1985, he attracted worldwide attention with his "honey-bee lens," especially designed to aid albinos and others with severely restricted fields of vision.

These days it's impossible for any printed list of visual aids to be up-to-date. A 1979 study of the partially sighted listed 130 optical and nonoptical aids for enhancing low vision. Since then the number of such aids has escalated. Each issue of the *Journal of Vision Rehabilitation* contains several pages of new low vision devices being introduced on the market and a special section on computer models adaptable for use by the partially sighted in offices, homes, libraries and schools.

The most common type of optical aid is the magnifier. It ranges from the small hand-held glass or plastic about the size of a silver dollar, through custom-designed magnifiers incorporated in conventional glasses to electronic systems that combine cameras with video screens capable of magnifying up to sixty times the original size of printed or typed documents.

For quick, short-term tasks like looking up phone numbers or reading menus in dimly lighted restaurants or checking price tags, small magnifiers, easy to carry in purse or pocket, are ideal for people with low vision. Larger hand-held magnifiers, though covering a greater area do not give so high a degree of magnification as the smaller ones, nor is the image so sharp. In this instance, larger is not necessarily better. Most of these larger magnifiers are heavy and hard to hold for any length of time, a decided handicap for people who may have arthritis or unsteady hands. Preferred by many readers are small magnifiers on circular stands that move easily across a page. Alternatives to these types of magnifiers are prescription magnifiers (telescopes, prisms, microscopes) or a combination of optic aids custom-designed for special tasks such as magnifiers used in microsurgery.

Telescopes designed to help people see distant objects or situations more clearly may be hand held or incorporated in glasses, or clipped to the top rim of glasses to boost the sight in one eye. The latter, known as jewelers' loupes, help the partially sighted "pull up" images in a limited field such as signatures, numerals on currency, or items on credit card statements.

For viewing street signs and numbers, watching sports events, or assessing traffic flow, many people with partial sight select hand-held telescopes. The lens prescription is for the "better eye" and most of these telescopes have a focusing mechanism. When not in use, they can be carried in a purse or pocket or suspended around the neck by a cord.

What is called a "full-diameter telescope," also designed for distance, is restricted to use when the wearer is stationary, that is, seated in a theater, ball park, at home watching TV, or in church. The telescope itself, set in a plastic eyeglass lens, is lightweight and convenient to wear. Though primarily for distance viewing, these telescopes can be converted into aids for close work with a reading lens over the telescopic lenses.

Telescopes designed specifically for reading and near tasks give the wearer a greater working distance than is possible with a reading cap of the same power. Instead of being mounted in the upper part of a conventional eyeglass lens, these telescopes are usually mounted low in the lens and angled downward in line with the normal reading position of the eyes. Without interfering with general seeing, the telescope is ready for near tasks, making it useful to secretaries, computer operators, students, electricians and others whose jobs involve "near" viewing.

Dr. Samuel M. Genensky, director of the Center for the Partially Sighted in Santa Monica, California, a pioneer in low vision services, and visually impaired himself, makes a strong case for the use of binoculars by the partially sighted. Blind in one eye and with severe sight loss in the other, Dr. Genensky uses binoculars extensively and advocates them for those with macular degeneration and other visual disorders. Eye doctors, he has found, do not usually favor binoculars for their partially sighted patients on the ground that those aids are too big, too heavy, and too conspicuous, an attitude Dr. Genensky says is common among clinicians and others with normal sight who can't imagine themselves using binoculars in public. Street use of binoculars does not have the social acceptance of crutches, even though these two types of aid serve a similar purpose—helping people get about conveniently and safely.

Dr. Genensky uses binoculars for reading street signs and seeing traffic lights, viewing chalkboards, watching scenery from a moving vehicle or television at home, and finding objects that have fallen to the floor or have been otherwise "visually misplaced." With their high magnification and large viewing area, binoculars are "excellent adjuncts to smaller optical systems such as telescopic aids," according to Dr. Genensky.

For near vision only, microscope spectacles (high-power magnifying lenses incorporated in prescription eyeglasses) are perhaps the easiest aids for prolonged

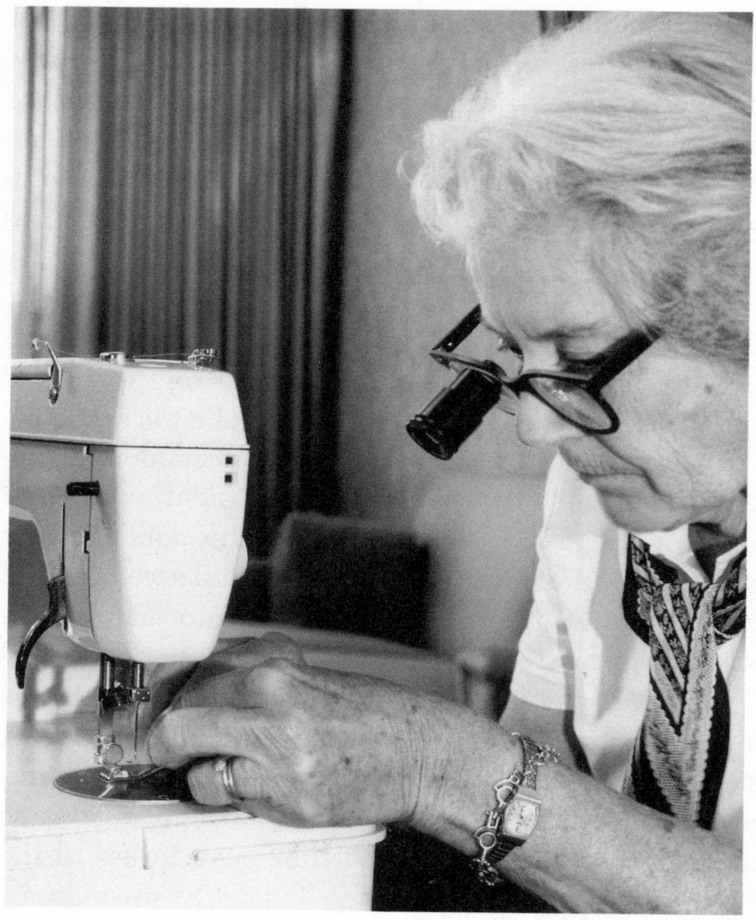

A telescopic lens enables this woman to use a sewing machine. (EYE RESEARCH INSTITUTE OF RETINA FOUNDATION)

reading and writing and for reading instructions on medicine bottles, examining stamps, or doing needlework. A drawback to microscopes is that, unless a person's distance prescription is incorporated, acuity is blurred when the wearer looks up from near tasks, sometimes causing dizziness, even nausea. But these microscopes are lightweight and "cosmetically acceptable," an important consideration in selecting any optical aid.

Weight is especially to be taken into account when prescribing optical aids for the elderly. Many older people cannot tolerate the heavy frames that support some telescopic and other aids. Even though prescription lenses give them the best possible visual acuity, the discomfort of the aid may be intolerable. Though they have already bought the aid, despite its cost, they may discard it and not return to the clinic for a replacement. One way clinics avoid this failure in the treatment program is to lend optical aids to patients for a trial period.

One low vision specialist told me, "When a patient is in a euphoric state over the almost magical improvement an aid gives his sight, he may not feel the weight on his nose, but after a week or two, it may be insupportable. When that happens, we make adjustments, sometimes compromises and trade-offs. To an elderly person it may be more important to sacrifice some sharpness of image for a comfortable aid."

An optical aid that is the target of much legislative and professional debate is the *bioptic telescope.* The question is whether drivers whose impaired vision can be improved by a bioptic telescope up to 20/40 acuity, the optical baseline for driver's licenses in most states, can qualify for driver permits. In an aging population marked by widespread visual impairments and dependent in many areas on private transportation, the need

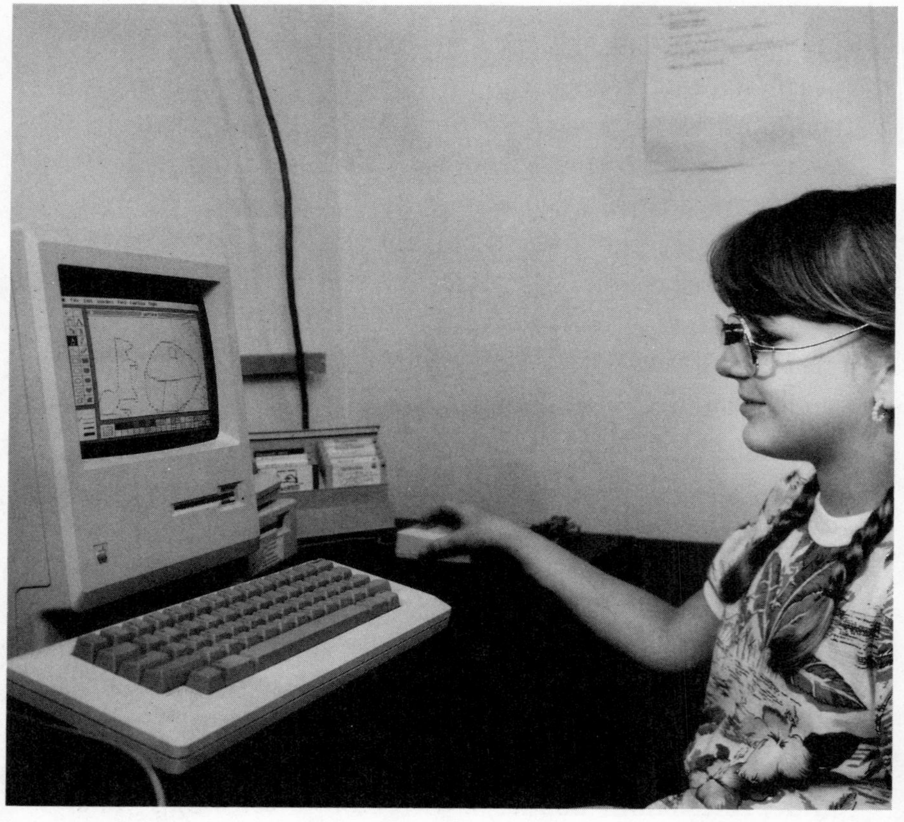

Visually impaired child using a computer with the aid of a small telescopic lens.
(EYE RESEARCH INSTITUTE OF RETINA FOUNDATION)

to reconcile legal and social demands has reached a critical stage. In 1985, some fourteen states licensed drivers whose low vision had been brought up to 20/40 acuity with bioptic telescopes.

Mounted in the top part of regular eyeglasses, these telescopes give the wearer greatly enhanced visual acuity for distance, yet when looking through the lower part of the glasses, the wearer sees a full field of vision with normal distance judgment.

"We have two models of bioptic aids," explains Richard Feinbloom, director of Designs for Vision Company and son of its founder, William Feinbloom. "One of the models was designed to improve the looks of the aids when that is a major consideration to wearers, especially to teenagers. The better-looking aid loses something in the size and brightness of the area being viewed, but that is one of the trade-offs that often have to be considered in selecting low vision aids."

But when a bioptic aid is the determining factor in keeping a job, appearance is of small consequence. A patient who lived in a state that sanctioned licensing drivers who wore bioptic aids was losing his central vision. As his sight had deteriorated, his regular glasses did not enable him to pass the vision test for a driver's permit. Since he was living on the outskirts of a small town and working in a plant thirty miles away, his problem was to get from his house to the town, where a car pool gathered for the drive to the plant. That four-mile drive from his house to town threatened his job.

During my visit to the Feinbloom clinic, I was permitted to accompany him and his trainer on a drive through suburban streets when he was being trained in using bioptic telescopes. Wearing his bioptic aid, he sat next to the trainer who drove the car. Prompted by questions ("Name of next street?" "Status of traffic light in next block?"), the patient, shifting his eyes from the telescopic lenses to his regular lenses in the lower part of the spectacles, sighted street signs and read the names aloud, then through his distance lenses he gave a running commentary on the flow of traffic, cars entering intersections, pedestrians crossing streets.

When we returned to the clinic, the trainer explained to me that this patient, after returning home, would wear his bioptic glasses (not while driving) for three months to get used to them and to coordinating eye movements essential for their use. Then he would spend another three months of practice with the aid while riding in a car as a passenger. Though he had been driving for years with regular glasses, he was advised—as are all other patients trained in using bioptics for driving—to take a course in driver training while wearing the bioptic telescopes.

The debate over whether drivers wearing bioptic telescopes should be given drivers' licenses is likely to continue for years. Results of studies are conflicting, some finding that these drivers have excellent safety records, others raising questions about the performance rating. One finding that seems conclusive is that the performance of drivers wearing bioptic telescopes is better if they live in small communities where they are familiar with the streets, traffic signs, the general environment, and hazardous conditions in all weathers and seasons.

A friend who wore bioptic telescopes for driving during the period when his sight was deteriorating told me that in retrospect he realizes dangers he couldn't acknowledge when his dependence on a car warped his

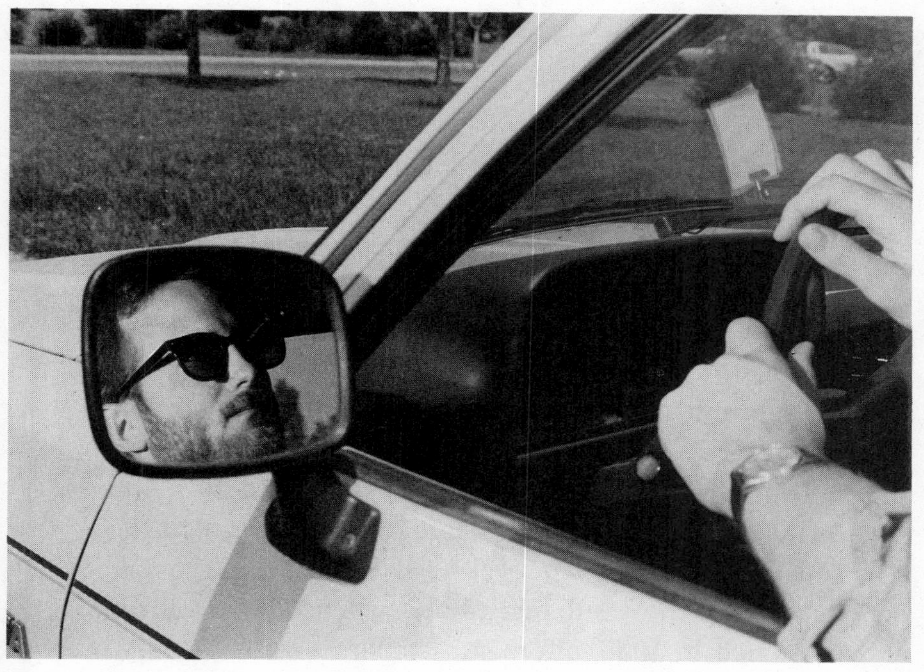

Driver using bioptic telescopic aid implanted in his regular glasses practices driving under supervision of instructor. (PHOTO COURTESY OF OPTOMETRY, UNIVERSITY OF HOUSTON, TEXAS)

judgment. He now feels that highway traffic, the speed, the plethora of signs on highways, the demands on the eye to shift constantly from distance to intermediate, to near are simply too stressful for an impaired visual system to cope with successfully. Others challenge this conclusion. The resolution of the debate may have to wait for the development of a visual aid that somehow reconciles optical needs with the exigencies of driving in today's high-speed traffic.

Accessory Aids

Accessory Aids is a term that includes homemaking aids, illumination controls, large print, leisure-activity aids, reading and writing aids. Broad as those categories are, they cannot encompass the plethora of nonoptical aids being produced commercially for the partially sighted, a recently discovered market. Coming out of the low vision network—self-help groups, publications and reports—are ingenious suggestions for solving everyday problems encountered by the partially sighted.

Best known among accessory aids are large-type books, including Bibles, magazines, and a special edition of *The New York Times.* The first large print book club, the Doubleday Large Print Home Library, launched in 1985, offers subscribers a wide variety of current best-sellers in fiction and nonfiction, including mysteries, biographies and how-to books in hardcover editions at reasonable cost and easy-to-read enlarged type. Some typewriters and photocopiers come with attachments for producing oversize type. Making out a check so a bank will accept it is one of the small, frustrating problems for people who can't see well. To help them with that problem are typescopes, black plastic overlays with sections cut out for the spaces to be filled in with dates, amount, name of recipient, and signature. These typescopes can be purchased at agencies for the partially sighted or through catalogs of low vision aids. But homemade versions are easily made using black paper and a razor. I use a version of the typescope for proofreading. Like most writers, I have trouble proofreading my typing. Though we may see the words and letters clearly enough, we tend to proofread not with our eyes, but with a kind of inner ear, reading for sense and style, and see not what is there but what we expect to see. Adding to the proofreading problem, "writer's tension" interferes with visual acuity. As a proofreading aid, I cut a space in a piece of black paper showing only one typed line, a device that by focusing my mind on the words helps me see them.

Glare from glossy paper can be reduced with an overlay of clear yellow plastic. This overlay not only cuts glare but makes the print darker. Another device, especially helpful for reading typed or printed materials is the Giant Magnifier, an 8½-by-11-inch piece of clear specially molded plastic that, when held a few inches above a typed or printed page, increases type size four times.

When one is tired, overwrought or distracted by a

neighbor's TV, concentrating on reading puts an added strain on the eye/brain visual system. A simple little device to rein in a wandering mind is the pointer. In medieval times, monks used them when reading manuscripts, moving the pointer from line to line. Today pointers called *yads* are used in synagogues for reading the Torah, not only to keep the reader's place but to prevent fingers from defiling the sacred manuscript. After learning about *yads,* I applied the "pointer principle" to my own reading, using something not so elaborate and precious as the *yads* in museum collections, but serviceable for keeping my place when engaged in heavy-duty research reading and speeding up my reading time. My pointer is a manicurist's cuticle stick.

Electronic Visual Aids

"Computers are going to become a common aid in low vision," predicts Dr. Gregory L. Goodrich, research psychologist at the Western Blind Rehabilitation Center, Veterans Administration Medical Center, in Palo Alto, California. Dr. Goodrich has been conducting studies of electronic aids for maximizing residual vision since the late 1970s, when their potential captured the imagination of researchers in the field of low vision. And, it should be added, about the same time many high-tech industries discovered the specialized market of partially sighted consumers.

Developments in computer technology occur so rapidly—new video machines, new applications of computers and word processors for the blind and partially sighted, the host of systems that transform standard computers into talking machines of extraordinary versatility—that it's almost impossible to keep up with them. Dr. Goodrich, who reports on these developments regularly in the *Journal of Vision Rehabilitation,* admits to the difficulty of providing up-to-date information about available electronic visual aids, let alone evaluating their efficacy for the partially sighted as manufacturers constantly improve the electronic hardware and develop innovative ways of adapting computers to the needs of the growing market among the partially sighted.

Most electronic visual aids are actually sophisticated magnifiers, the polished beryl and crystal used by scholars in ancient times raised to incredibly higher power by technology.

According to Dr. Goodrich, the idea of applying television technology to the problems of the visually impaired was first proposed in an article in the *American Journal of Ophthalmology* in 1959, an idea that was seized on by the gifted innovator Dr. Samuel M. Genensky, who developed closed-circuit television (CCTV) and training programs essential to the use of this electronic system as a visual aid.

CCTV is one of the most widely used visual systems in schools, offices and libraries, and in the homes of business people and professionals. The system uses a mounted camera that focuses downward on a page (a typewritten letter, page of a book or magazine, handwritten note, newspaper clipping) and transmits the image electronically to an adjacent television screen where letters are magnified to the specifications of the user. Some CCTVs magnify as much as sixty times, enabling children and adults who have only a tiny part of usable retina for reading.

A drawback to CCTV and other electronic magnifying systems is that the larger the letters the fewer the words on the screen, which slows reading and tests patience. But for those who could not read without them, these magnifying systems are tolerated psychologically as users learn to read faster. Adding to their versatility are special attachments, such as scanning adapters for viewing blackboards, and attachments for typewriters and adding machines.

Vtek (formerly Visualtek) was among the first companies to adapt the CCTV concept commercially to the needs of the partially sighted. In 1985, it was the largest company producing a variety of electronic visual devices used in offices, classrooms, libraries, and in retirement and private homes. Vtek systems not only magnify electronically, but at the same time sharpen the print image on the screen.

The Vtek Voyager model includes a closed circuit camera above a small platform that holds materials to be read and transmitted to the TV display screen. This standard model magnifies up to forty times the original size of letters to be read. The Voyager XL has a larger screen and magnification power up to sixty times.

These electronic magnifiers are a boon to partially sighted children in classrooms, to students and career people with poor vision. They also aid rare-book and manuscript scholars whose normal vision is severely strained by continuous reading of ancient and medieval scripts. Not to be overlooked are partially sighted collectors of coins and stamps, who are enabled to con-

the rail.
Alec saw the man's
being lowered.
he was climbing
into the boat!
man lost his
VISUALTEK

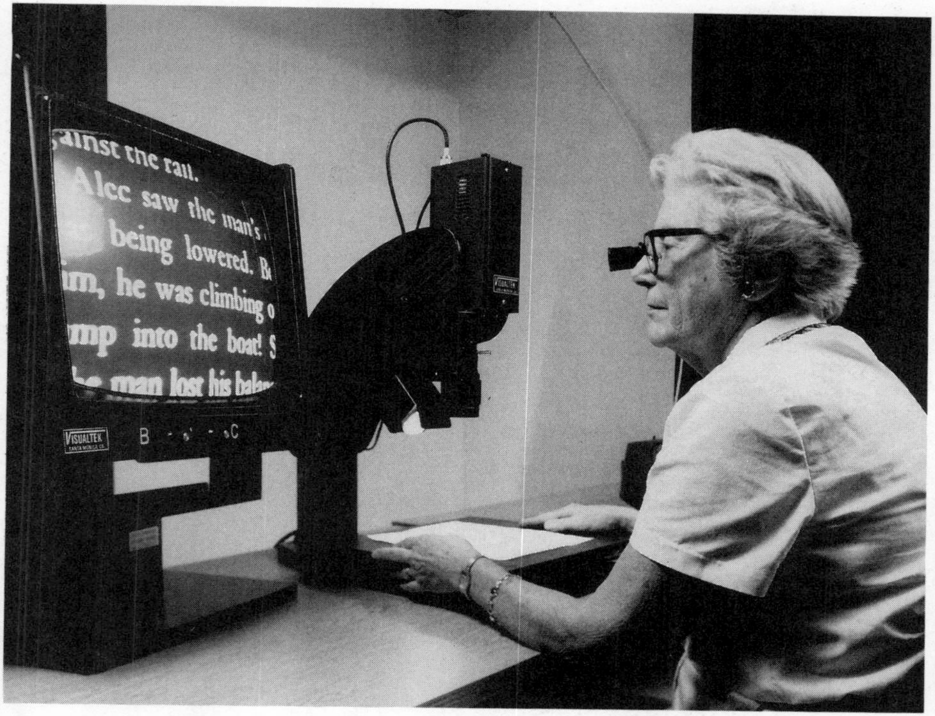

The combination of a TV screen with magnified letters, a camera that photographs the printed page and a telescopic aid enables this woman to read.
(EYE RESEARCH INSTITUTE OF RETINA FOUNDATION)

tinue their hobbies with that extra magnification and clarity provided by electronic visual devices.

Vtek's Typing Aid System provides a free-standing camera that peers over the typewriter and sends a magnified image to an adjacent video screen, enabling

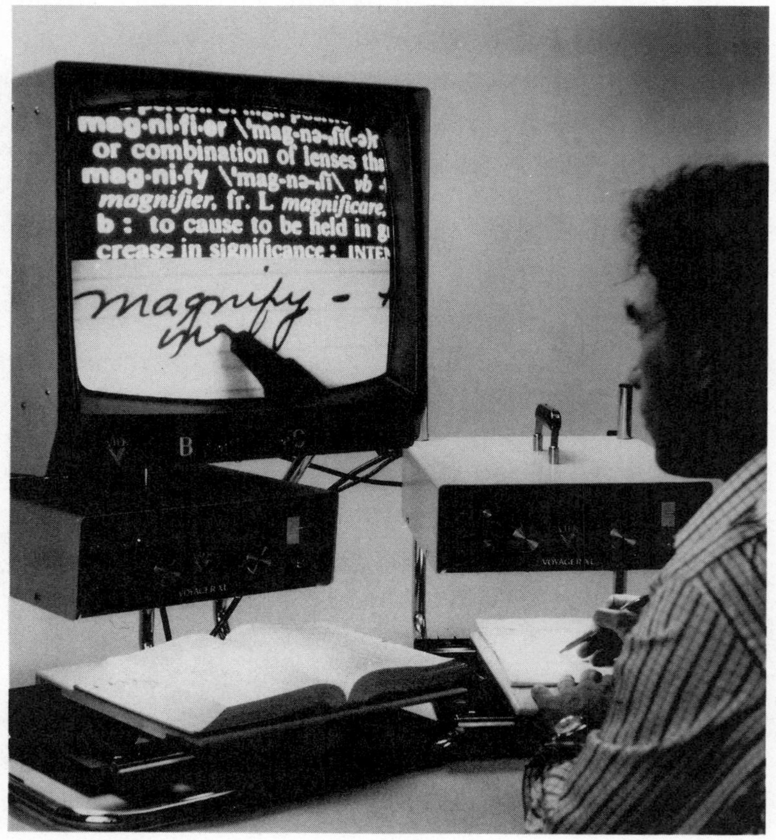

A TV-and-camera device enables this visually handicapped man to read and write. (PHOTO COURTESY OF VTEK)

the typist to see copy as it is being typed and to proofread and make corrections.

An electronic reading aid that came on the market in the early 1980s is Viewscan, a portable magnifying system developed for the partially sighted. Viewscan fits into a briefcase and is designed to withstand the stress of rigorous travel. To operate this machine, the reader holds a miniature camera about the size of a cigarette lighter and moves it on rollers across a page, producing a greatly magnified image on the Viewscan display screen. Besides its magnification, Viewscan's advantages are its light weight (8 pounds) and portability.

To mention one more electronic viewing aid: the Optiscope's illuminated enlarger system Model C, a compact unit weighing fourteen pounds. One of its advantages is that students with low vision can use it to study the same textbooks used by their normally sighted classmates. Its movable platform holds books, magazines, newspapers, letters, photographs in black and white or in full color, drawings and maps. The fourteen-inch screen of this self-contained unit has brightness control by the viewer, a decided asset for those whose light tolerance and adaptability often varies from day to day.

Computer terminals, separate units connected to a "host" computer, are another electronic magnifying device. One such is the Apollo Computer Terminal System that, according to Dr. Goodrich, is so easy to use that even a novice can master it in an hour or two. With magnification adjustable up to letters slightly

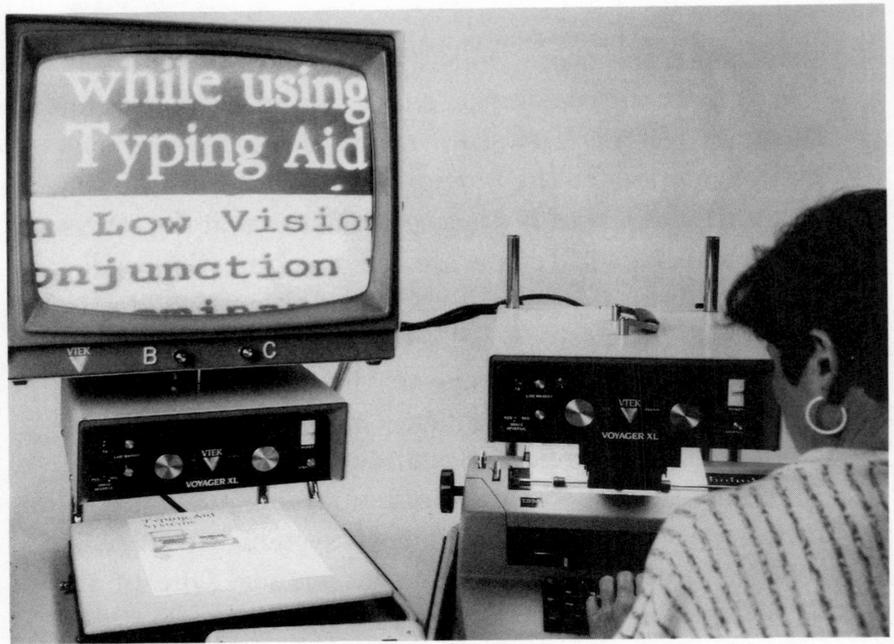

A TV-and-camera combination attached to a typewriter makes typing possible for this woman.
(PHOTO COURTESY OF VTEK)

more than four inches high, this system is used in a variety of work and educational settings, libraries, and other institutions that have computer systems. But, warns Dr. Goodrich, buyers of terminals for use with computers should make certain that terminals and computers are compatible. "A common frustrating experience among computer users," says Dr. Goodrich, "is buying equipment that doesn't work with what you need it to work with."

Dr. Goodrich advises potential buyers of electronic

vision-enhancing equipment to shop around and compare models, always relating the machines' capabilities to the buyers' own specific needs (such as what they want the computer to do for them). It's difficult to determine cost-effectiveness of these electronic visual aids. What it comes down to is how much a machine is worth that gets you where you want to go. These days people spend from $10,000 to $20,000 or more for cars to transport them from one place to another and usually have to borrow money to buy that mechanized transportation. For thousands of partially sighted men and women it may be equally important to spend several hundred or several thousand dollars (even if they have to get a bank loan) for a device that enables them to continue careers in which they have already heavily invested time, effort and money.

Dr. Otis Stephens, professor of political science at the University of Tennessee and vice-president of the American Council of the Blind, says that the new technology

> is rapidly closing the communications gap that for generations has posed a major problem, especially in education and employment. With the development of personal computers and rapid improvements in word processing, it is now possible for the blind and partially sighted to prepare and edit material in final form and to have direct access to the printed page. Perhaps the greatest advantage of all is that one need not have specialized knowledge of computers to make effective use of them. Advances during the past few years or so are probably comparable in importance to the invention of braille itself.

Dr. Stephens, who is legally blind, uses a system that combines a personal computer with a VersaBraille unit with an electronic keyboard that enables him to record the equivalent of 400 pages of braille information on one sixty-minute cassette tape. Dr. Stephens says, "I can not only store hundreds of pages of braille notes on a single cassette tape, but what is more helpful to me is being able to edit and proofread my own written reports, manuscripts and course outlines without having to rely on a sighted reader."

Because of limited demand, many of the new electronic aids to viewing are not mass-produced, resulting in high unit costs, which in turn prevent the market from expanding. "Though some modest price reductions have taken place," Dr. Stephens says, "major reductions won't occur until the technology is used by many more people. It's certain that several hundred thousand, if not a million, blind and partially sighted people in the United States could make effective use of these new electronic devices. The American Council of the Blind has been using many methods to focus attention on these devices and is exploring new ways of publicizing the latest developments and making the new technology readily available to more people who could benefit from it."

Though technically not vision enhancers, reading machines are so valuable to those with severe visual disorders that they are included in this section on electronic aids. Their great value to those with defective sight is that students and professional people can select precisely the information they need whether in a book, professional journal, magazine, newspaper or newsletter. Talking books, especially those distributed by the Library of Congress, though an invaluable source of information and pleasure to thousands of the visually handicapped, rarely contain special reference material needed by students, scientists, financial experts and others.

The Kurzweil Reading Machine, first marketed in 1977, uses a small computer-controlled camera that scans lines of print and recognizes each letter. Using spaces between words to define a set of letters as a word, the computer draws on its memory for rules of English grammar and pronunciation (several *thousand* rules) to determine how to say the word then activates the voice synthesizer. If the voice does not sound like that of your favorite newscaster, consider what it has gone through to come out even with a semblance of the human voice. I am told by users of the Kurzweil Reading Machine and other computers with voice synthesizers that one gets used to the sound of mechanized voices. But improvements are on the way as industry and commercial establishments use synthetic voices in elevators, supermarkets, and in robots that skitter around factories or give sales pitches at trade association conventions. Kurzweil and other producers of synthetic voice machines are constantly improving diction, inflection, timbre and tone of these disembodied voices.

The changing nature of technology, according to Dr. Goodrich, is something we must learn to live with.

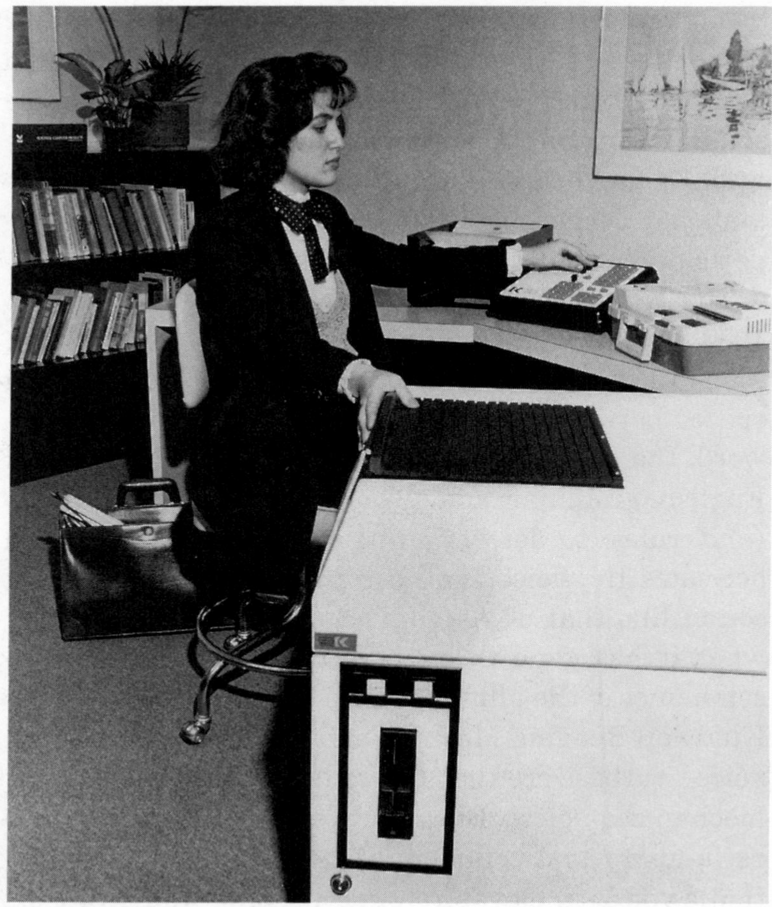

The Kurzweil Reading Machine converts printed or typewritten texts into synthetic voice sounds. The machine operator places the text on the glass surface of the scanner and activates the reading voice system by pressing buttons on the separate control panel. The speed, volume and pitch of the voice can be adjusted, and the machine can be directed to repeat material and to read punctuation and capitalization. (KURZWEIL COMPUTER PRODUCTS, INC.)

That's especially true in regard to computers. And the fact that today's tool may be out of date tomorrow does not mean that we should not use today's tool. With computers playing an ever-increasing role in our lives, it's evident that the visually impaired person's needs for computer skills are no different from the needs of people with normal vision in business, schools, and in the numerous situations that require access to information. Without such access to computers, the visually impaired as a group will be more disadvantaged than they have been at any time in the past, which will only compound their problems.

Voice Indexing

In the 1970s, when national attention was being focused on the handicapped, with special emphasis on access to buildings and public transportation, James G. Chandler was leading his own crusade for what he called "intellectual access" for the blind and partially sighted. A retired reference librarian at the University of Maryland, Chandler, though sighted, had learned braille in preparation for volunteer work with the blind. His library experience and volunteer work convinced him that, though physical access for the handicapped solved numerous problems, there was another type of access to be addressed, namely access to information. The blind and thousands of partially sighted had to rely on sighted helpers to provide them with reference materials they could not find in books, reports, and recorded notes of lectures in college classes and meetings. They could not look up words in dictionaries or keep track of social and business engagements on personal calendars. To find a particular recipe in a recorded cookbook, they had to play the tape until they came to the recipe.

Though an enormous amount of information was being taped by professional organizations, publishers, lecturers and other individuals, finding a particular passage on a cassette was a slow, cumbersome and uncertain process compared with the page-flipping done by the sighted. Chandler points out:

> The sighted are aided by descriptive chapter titles, boldface sub-headings, italics, marginal notes and other visual cues. Reference books, dictionaries, encyclopedias, and a host of compendia of facts that are not intended to be read in one long gulp are almost worthless when taped without effective finding devices.
>
> I was convinced there must be a simple, inexpensive and reasonably prompt way of finding information already taped, but the look-up potential of this equipment had scarcely been explored. With absolutely no technical knowledge or skills, I began experimenting with simple tape-recording equipment until I made it index by the spoken word, making it possible for a person to locate a specific item on a tape just as a newspaper reader uses headlines to scan a page of newsprint.

One result of his concern about the "look-up" needs of the visually handicapped and his advocacy of voice indexing is that, with an acknowledgment to Chandler, the Library of Congress's National Library Service for the Blind and Physically Handicapped produced the first voice-indexed dictionary, recorded from Houghton Mifflin's *Concise American Heritage Dictionary.* Chandler himself has developed a voice-indexing system for use by individuals on 4-track and 2-track cassette recorders.

Voice indexing is a boon not only to the blind and partially sighted, but also to those with normal vision whose work involves extensive recording—journalists, scientists and writers. Much information I had taped at meetings or during interviews was frustratingly inaccessible without playing entire tapes until I learned Chandler's method of voice indexing using a 2-track recorder. Not one to keep information inaccessible, Chandler founded the nonprofit organization Voice Indexing for the Blind, Inc., which publishes lists of voice-indexed publications and an instruction manual for voice indexing on a 2-track cassette recorder. (See Appendix for address.)

Grateful as the partially sighted should be for the plethora of aids to help them see better and low vision specialists to assist them in maximizing the use of what vision they have, the partially sighted owe a debt to a group that in the long run will have an enormous impact on their visual efficiency—industrial market analysts who recently have discovered them, their needs, and their potential for profitability. This discovery is now spurring research, development and sales—good news for the partially sighted today and in the future.

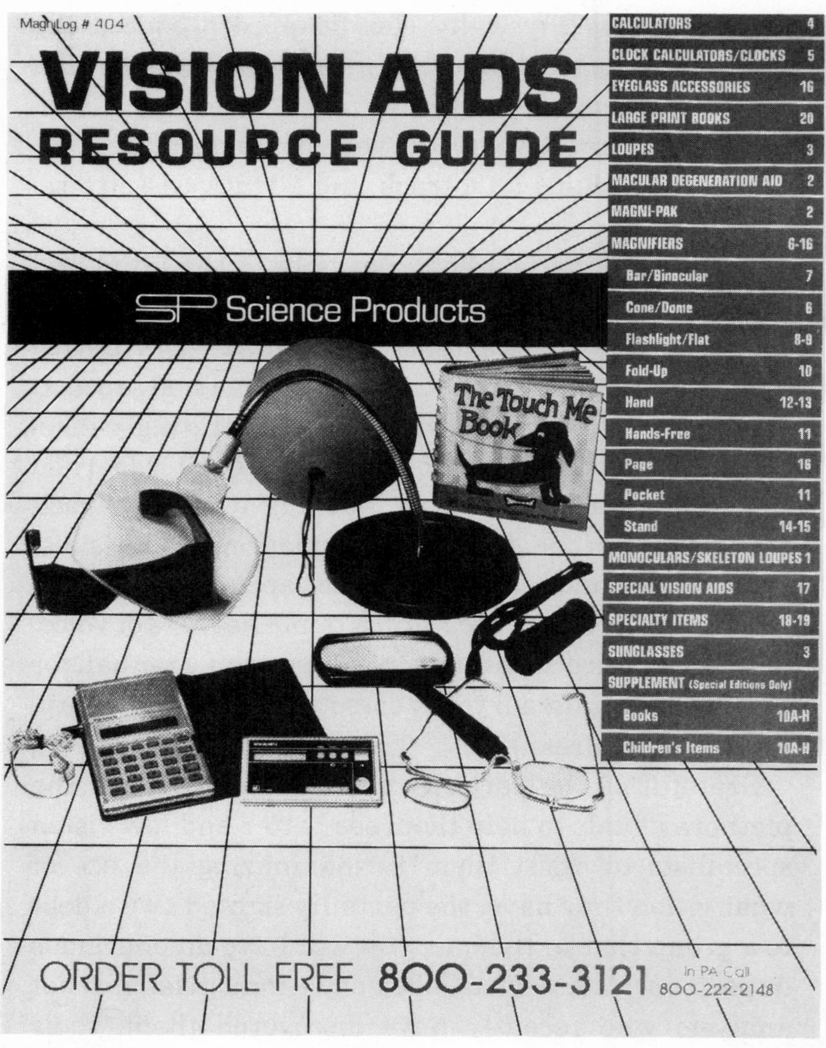

A catalog of visual aids, ranging from special calculators designed for the visually handicapped to loupes, monoculars and other specialty items. SCIENCE PRODUCTS

Training in Use of Aids

Whatever the type of aid, whether hand-held magnifiers, special lenses in conventional glasses, or electronic aids, instruction is essential for their efficient use. How long it will take a patient to learn to use an aid efficiently depends on the patient's intelligence, motivation, self-esteem and, in some instances, physical condition. Some elderly people, though strongly motivated, may be physically incapable of the sustained effort possible for younger, more robust patients. Most low vision clinics, to accommodate the frailties of elderly patients, pace the training series over several weeks.

When teaching a patient how to use an optical aid, the low vision specialist generally starts off by explaining the structure of the aid and how it will help the patient's vision, how to hold and focus the aid. If it's a hand-held magnifier, how to move it smoothly across lines and pages to reduce tension in the muscles of the hand. A reading stand may be advised for those who have difficulty holding books or other printed materials. Patients who will wear telescopic or microscopic lenses are taught how to scan written or typed pages and how to improve their reading speed. If they will use two or more aids for different types of tasks (near and far) they are instructed about the importance of maintaining the distance for which the aids have been prescribed. Patients with macular degeneration or other eye disorders that affect central vision usually require a great deal of practice in learning to substitute peripheral for central vision. But, as recounted in a previous chapter, *New York Times* reporter Robert Trumbull, using a special optical aid, mastered the technique of eccentric viewing in one sitting.

Electronic aids (CCTV, Vtek, Opticon and others) require more extensive training. Even before they start, some patients have to overcome "computer phobia," something quite common even among the sighted. But once patients understand the mechanics of the machines and learn to use them, they are likely to become addicted and to wonder how they ever managed without them. But these electronic aids, though some are portable, are primarily for sedentary users whose tasks are performed at desks or tables.

Training in using telescopic lenses, binoculars, or bioptics prescribed for distance viewing is usually supplemented by mobility training for getting about streets and buildings, spotting landmark cues, and avoiding lampposts and other frequently encountered obstacles on sidewalks, including other pedestrians, monitoring flow of traffic at intersections, and adjusting to different degrees of visibility in various weather conditions.

Important in training to use these distance aids is learning to adjust to distortions caused by the lenses or, with bioptics, learning quickly to shift the gaze from distance to close viewing. Some low vision clinics have mobility trainers who teach how to quickly shift the gaze from distance to close viewing. Clinics without such specialists refer patients to local agencies that provide mobility training or to professional instructors in private practice.

This chapter has given you some idea of the great variety of aids for enhancing vision. One reason many partially sighted people are unaware of the availability of this vast resource, according to the American Optometric Association, is that many aids are distributed primarily by organizations for the blind, a source that those who are not blind will not naturally turn to. But as more agencies for the blind give greater publicity to their services for the partially sighted, their resources for that special segment of the population will become better known.

In the Appendix of this book, you will find listed sources that provide optical, nonoptical, and accessory aids and catalogs of aids.

6

Adapting the Personal Environment

As vision deteriorates, the once familiar, safe household has a disconcerting way of developing hazards that didn't seem to exist before. Staircases that were once descended without looking down at all become perilous, one tread indistinguishable from another. Scatter rugs that one used to walk on surefootedly, slide from underneath. Tiled bathrooms, their light intensity once perfect for shaving or putting on make-up, develop a blinding glare. One is less likely to notice the dog or cat stretched out in pathways from one room to another. Tripping over invisible family pets is a common accident for the partially sighted, adding broken bones to an already crowded list of problems. Some people reluctantly get rid of pets they have difficulty seeing. But there are other solutions—an elderly woman, whose sight had deteriorated to the point where she kept tripping over the Siamese cat that blended into the gray living-room carpet, instead of getting rid of the cat as everyone advised, had the carpet dyed a deep reddish brown that contrasted with the silvery cat.

So much attention in low vision treatment programs focuses on the array of aids and training that others provide to help the visually impaired see better, that those with low vision seldom consider the many ways in which they can help themselves. There's not much we can do to change the visibility of the outside environment, but there is a great deal the visually handicapped can do to increase the visibility and safety of their homes, which often remain static over the years while declining vision requires changes. A succession of accidents, often minor, but sometimes disastrous, can be an early indication of declining sight and should be the signal for bringing the home into conformity with changing visual needs and living patterns.

The best way to start a home adaptation program is to begin with a survey. Take a fresh look at your house or apartment, viewing it critically as if seeing it for the first time and as objectively as a prospective buyer or renter. Think of it in terms of your present and future needs and physical capacities.

An assessment of the home visual environment should begin with that fundamental medium of sight: lighting. British lighting experts who assess lighting efficiency in homes of partially sighted residents report that increased illumination, type of light appropriate to activities, and proper location of light sources vastly improve visual ability. In some instances, after poor lighting has been corrected, some elderly people have been able to get along at home without using special optical aids.

Home lighting assessment is one of the many special services the British provide their partially sighted citizens, who are registered separately from the blind. If, for instance, a home lighting assessment indicates that a certain type of lamp is needed in a home and the partially sighted resident can't afford to pay for it, on authorization of an eye doctor, a public agency purchases the lamp. As a British official told me, compared to the cost of institutional care, assistance that enables those with impaired vision to stay in their homes makes good economic sense, not to mention what it means for those people to live independently in their own homes. Eye doctors could contribute significantly to the visual well-being of patients if, when advising them about optical aids, they stressed the importance of good home lighting. Rarely does it occur to patients that one cause of their visual deficiency could be inadequate, inappropriate lighting.

The survey of home lighting should include rooms, hallways, stairs (inside and outdoors), closets, storage areas, basements and attics, and relating the adequacy of lighting to the location of those areas, for instance, whether those areas get daylight from windows, are on the sunny side of the dwelling, or are windowless hallways. Not only should the location of areas be considered, but what goes on in them; the family social center requires entirely different lighting from that in the kitchen or home office.

A general guide for home lighting is to avoid pronounced differences in degree of light between areas. Going from a dark hall into the glare of a bathroom of white tiles and mirrors requires rapid adjustment for normal eyes, an adjustment that takes much longer for eyes impaired by age or defects. Most of us have experienced the disorientation of going from bright sunlight into a dark theater and trying to locate a seat with some dignity. Minimizing differences in degree of light between rooms can be accomplished with small, low-wattage bulbs set in baseboards to give diffused but efficient light at all times, especially in bedrooms, bathrooms, and at the tops of stairs.

Ideal home lighting combines good general lighting from fixtures in ceilings or on walls with focused lighting from table or floor lamps. Adequate lighting properly placed is one of the most inexpensive and effective ways of enhancing marginal vision. Home lighting experts stress not only the degree of light and the location of its source, but the importance of distance between light source and whatever a person is looking at. Reading by a ceiling light is not only hard on the eyes, but inefficient; the farther the light source from the task, the weaker the illumination.

Bright, reflected light from any shiny surfaces—a polished floor, bathroom tiles, white porcelain kitchen work space—is especially hard on aging eyes, because the pupils don't contract properly to shut out the excessive light. As glare can occur in any room in the house, it is something the home surveyor should look for and take measures to reduce.

Kitchens

A logical place to begin the home visibility assessment is the kitchen, where light intensity and location are of major importance, a place of hazards even for those with keen sight. People with low vision are probably the best-organized cooks in the world. If they weren't, few edible meals would come out of their kitchens. Not only must they cope with the usual hazards, but they have the added difficulty of finding food in the freezer, cutlery in drawers, a can or jar on a cabinet shelf, the right pan in a stack of pots and pans. Unless their work areas, drawers, cabinets, refrigerators and freezers are systematically organized and items are clearly identified (usually by coarsely textured, coded tape or by labels hand-printed in heavy black letters), partially sighted cooks spend more time looking for things than using them.

To fully sighted people it is a marvel that those with low vision manage to slice, chop and mix ingredients, and even cook gourmet meals and serve them attractively. But they do. My partially sighted acquaintances in the National Capital Citizens with Low Vision, mostly professionals in their thirties and forties, give some of the best supper parties I've ever attended. As hosts they seem less anxious than sighted hosts, possibly because they are so used to coping daily with their own special anxieties in jobs, getting about, shopping and all the things sighted people do so readily, that giving a party doesn't faze them in the least.

A first consideration in adapting the kitchen to impaired vision is the walls. There is no immutable rule that says kitchen walls should be white. Pastels are easier on the eyes. But walls should not be covered with glossy paint. It may be easy to keep clean, but the glare is troublesome to defective eyes.

The kitchen is one room in the house or apartment where fluorescent light is desirable and advantageous. Generally used more extensively in offices and industrial plants, fluorescent lighting is *worker* lighting, the preferred light source in commercial and public buildings because its light output is about four times that of incandescent lamps, it diffuses light over wide areas, and it radiates less heat (a factor in air-conditioned space). But for all that, it has aesthetic drawbacks. It distorts colors, washing out the red spectrum. And the stroboscopic flickering, even when apparently undetectable, has a fatiguing effect, according to safety studies in work places. As one low vision specialist says, fluorescent light and the elderly don't go well together.

Despite that, because most people don't spend the entire day in their kitchens, fluorescent lighting serves a good purpose there. Incandescent ceiling lights rarely provide bright enough light for cutting and chopping and mixing. Besides, they're apt to cast shadows on the work space, where unobstructed light is most needed. Strip fluorescent lights beneath cabinets and above the work area and sink dispel shadows and provide the needed bright light.

A simple, seldom-considered way of intensifying kitchen light is suggested by lighting experts: keep bulbs and light tubes clean and replace them when it's obvious from their dimming or flickering that they're losing power. Keeping light fixtures clean is important in any room, but special attention should be given to kitchen lights, which accumulate smoke and grease. According to experts, the efficiency of dirty light bulbs and tubes can be reduced by as much as 50 percent.

Contrast in any room, hall or stairway does wonders to sharpen visual images, something especially true in the kitchen, where visibility and safety are so closely related. A reversible slicing board, light on one side and dark on the other, provides contrast for cutting meats, fish, and vegetables. The edges of white or light-colored mixing bowls have a way of fading into a white surface, causing misjudgments when pouring ingredients or cracking eggs. A solution to this vexation is to place a piece of dark, nonskid plastic beneath the light-colored bowl.

The ingenuity of partially sighted cooks is boundless. A suggestion that a partially sighted friend gave me for this book is to keep in a kitchen cabinet some basic first-aid equipment: compresses and Band-Aids. If a person with impaired vision cuts himself or herself, it may be a long way to the medicine cabinet; unnecessary panic can be avoided if aid is within arm's reach.

Cookbooks now come in large print, but for those who have difficulty reading even large type, cookbooks are now available on cassettes, some of them voice-indexed.

Stove dials with raised numerals are on the market, but one partially sighted woman solved her problems of setting the dial correctly by taping on the dial toothpicks, broken at different lengths, the longest piece at 350 degrees, and decreased lengths for marking increased temperatures. VISTA (Visually Impaired Secretarial/Transcribers Association) puts out a voice-indexed cassette of ingenious household hints primarily for the visually impaired, but useful for the sighted too.

An indispensable kitchen aid is the timer with large numerals, an alerter for the "doneness" of food and a reminder to turn off the stove. Timers are also reminders to preoccupied cooks to get ready for appointments. People with low vision generally need extra time to do things that sighted people can do with dispatch.

Family Rooms

When we visualize the family room we tend to see it as a stage setting: sofas, chairs and tables arranged in ensembles as if ready to be photographed for an interior-decoration magazine, everything in perfect order except that there are no people on our imaginary set. Unless furniture is in a museum, roped off with velvet cords and "Please do not touch" signs, it is used by family and guests who actively engage in talking, reading, nibbling, drinking, watching television, and moving things about. Not many living rooms have furniture bolted to the floor as did that of Baynard Kendrick's blind detective, Captain Duncan Maclain, who moved about his penthouse with quick sure steps, confident that each piece of furniture was in its accustomed place, firmly fixed to the floor. That arrangement did well for the blind detective, but most partially sighted people don't go to that extreme. There is, however, much they can do to increase the visibility of furniture and, indeed, of the entire room, its openness and sense of order.

Without being bolted to the floor, furniture can be arranged so there are no major surprises for members of the family who see poorly. To be able to move about a room with ease and safety fosters a sense of well-being and confidence. Dr. DeWitt Stetten, now that he is blind, says that coffee tables are the abomination of life. His bruised shinbones attest to painful encounters with the corners of those obstacles. Some hosts are embarrassed about calling a partially sighted guest's attention to low tables, protruding legs of chairs, ottomans, or a friendly dog soliciting a pat on the head. But hard-of-seeing guests much prefer warnings to bruises or falls and weeks in a cast. Better than warnings is removal of obstacles before guests arrive. People with impaired vision are more concerned about making spectacles of themselves in strange settings than in having their disability acknowledged. This fear of making a scene in the presence of sighted people is one that keeps many visually impaired people home.

In adapting rooms to accommodate the declining vision of family members, things to consider besides arranging furniture to increase its visibility are the color and textures of upholstery or slip covers. Textures that reflect light in different ways provide clues to the location of sofas and chairs. A chair cover that blends with the carpet is destined to confuse someone with poor sight. It doesn't matter that the person has sat on that chair numerous times, in moments of stress or dim light an accident can happen. Not many of us sit down with the assurance of Queen Victoria, who never looked, but simply sat, confident that someone in attendance would make certain that she and the seat of the chair came together simultaneously.

A room in which carpet and furniture are the same color may look interesting in a magazine photograph, but it is not a practical decor for anyone with poor eyesight. Without contrast, things blend confusingly together, and in diffused lighting no shadows accentuate furniture and other objects. But too many different patterns in rugs, upholstery and draperies can create visual chaos. Home decorating to enhance vision means an uncluttered image, bold but simple patterns in textiles, strong contrast between walls and furniture and between walls and doors either by outlining the doors or giving them visibility with contrasting wood or paint. Glass doors are a serious hazard and should be clearly marked with tape or stenciled stripes. I once saw a man with perfect sight walk through the plate-glass door of a clinic. His normal vision had been temporarily impaired by panic—he had just been told that he had cancer.

In no other room of the house is there so much latitude in type, location and direction of lighting as in the family room. Older couples usually have their favorite chairs and individual lighting. Younger adults and their children in the common room generally prefer overhead and wall lighting, especially when conversation is the main activity. For individual lighting, the type of lamp recommended by most lighting experts for those with low vision is the flexible-arm or gooseneck lamp that can be adjusted for distance from the task at hand whether it's reading, handwork, playing cards or other table games.

It's interesting that only certain lamps are recommended to help people see better. You might think that was the purpose of all lamps and lighting, but such is not the fact. How many advertisements for lamps say anything about improving visual efficiency? Rather, the ads stress the design of the lamp—the artistry of a Japanese jar converted into a table lamp, style of an Art Deco floor lamp, a cluster of tubular lamp shades that focus light straight down on the floor. It would be a boon to the population at large if designers of lamps knew a bit about the dynamics of vision and the prevalence of subnormal vision among Americans over fifty years of age.

Dining Areas

The biggest problem the partially sighted have with dining is being able to see the food. White china on white or very light tablecloths and place mats gives no definition to the edges of plates, cups and saucers. Food gets pushed onto the cloth or mat, cream is poured into the saucer, and sugar misses its mark. To avoid these gaucheries, contrasting colors should be used at the table, dark china on light tablecloths or mats or vice versa. Glassware should be in contrasting colors or rimmed with a colored stripe. Colorful and attractive as they may be, checked, striped or floral patterns in tablecloths and place mats create another visual trap for those with low vision.

Basic to seeing well in the dining area is strong illuminance either from a chandelier over the table or from wall sconces. Candlelight is anathema to diners with defective vision. And it does not enhance the beauty of anyone who wears glasses.

Busy patterns in dining-area carpets or linoleum do not provide strong enough contrast for chairs for safe seating. Scientists at Northwestern University in studies of aging eyes found that at certain distances, older people needed three times as much contrast to see patterns as clearly as did younger people taking part in the studies. In their report, the scientists pointed out that measurements of contrast sensitivity would not have showed up in standard eye examinations. It is only recently that contrast has been recognized as one of the most important aids to enhancing visibility of the environment. Contrast not only makes objects more visible, but stimulates the eye/brain visual system to perform more efficiently. It's one of the ironies of our time that while the military spends millions of dollars figuring out ways to make troops and armored vehicles invisible in battle, low vision experts, lighting engineers and designers are just as busy (on smaller budgets) applying the concepts of contrast to heighten visibility in homes and work places to aid those with impaired sight.

Stairways

"When partially sighted people encounter a flight of stairs they frequently find that they cannot distinguish the individual steps," says Dr. Samuel M. Genensky in an article in *Building Operating Management.* Partially sighted himself, Dr. Genensky knows all too well the sensation experienced by a person with impaired vision when he confronts a flight of stairs. "These stairways and steps look like a surface or mass that lacks any distinguishable markings or contours. This is particularly true when the stairs lead to a lower level." For both inside and outside stairs, Dr. Genensky recommends marking the leading edge of each step on both the runner and the riser with a strip of paint or a strip of nonskid material that runs the width of the step.

Railings should be painted a color that contrasts with that of the steps and background. In the house, there should be a baseboard light at the top and bottom of the flight of steps. Overhead lights at the top of the steps cast the shadow of the person descending, making the descent even more perilous. Sometimes the very fear of making a misstep and falling causes elderly people to waver, tilt off balance, and fall as they feared they would. Every precaution should be taken to minimize the inherent dangers of navigating stairs, including using solid-colored carpets and textures that won't catch the rough edges of worn heels.

Bedrooms

The bedroom is a special place in most homes. Not only a room for sleeping, it is a private place, a room for making love, for secret talks out of earshot of the rest of the family and, at times of emotional turmoil, a refuge.

Arranging furniture in a bedroom doesn't give the home decorator much leeway. Everything else in the room must be subordinate to the bed or beds. The main visual problems in the bedroom stem from lighting, its intensity and placement, and from pathways in and out of the room.

In general, there should be a shielded ceiling light to illuminate the entire room. Light switches should be handy to doors and either the illuminated type that lights when the switch is in the "off" position, or of a color that strongly contrasts with that of the walls or outlined with a contrasting border. Illuminated switches are beacons, orientation points for people getting up in the night. Small, dim, continuously lighted bulbs in baseboards near bedroom doors and in the bathroom help night walkers safely find their way. In adapting the bedroom to diminished vision, be sure that any unanchored scatter rugs have nonskid mats beneath them. Of foremost importance are unobstructed pathways to doors.

Not even the experts agree about individual lighting for reading in bed. Some suggest a shaded lamp centered over the headboard; others suggest a lamp on a bedside table. If the table is between twin beds, light from the lamp should impartially serve both beds and the lamp should have dual switches. One thing the experts do agree on is that the bedside lamps should have sturdy bases to prevent their being knocked over by half-asleep people fumbling for the switch. Some travelers with low vision wisely pack a battery lamp to augment the notoriously dim bedside lamps in hotels, something even keenly sighted travelers complain about.

The same principle of organization that enables the partially sighted to function well in the kitchen applies to bedrooms that serve as dressing rooms and storage areas for clothes and accessories. Those whose sight has been long in the decline have worked out systems for arranging clothes and accessories for easy, quick retrieval. Needless to say, there should be a bright closet light activated by a light switch. Some partially sighted people organize their clothes by seasons and type of apparel, sports, business and dress clothes separated, sometimes using plastic cleaners' bags as readily identified dividers.

In households of the partially sighted the old adage, "A place for everything and everything in its place," has special significance. It can be a matter of survival.

Telephones

Sighted people dial phone numbers almost unconsciously (one reason for so many wrong numbers), but people with impaired vision have to pay strict attention to the numerals and usually need some sort of visual aid. A time-saving device that can be either an adjunct to or replacement for the phone directory is a personal directory, listing in large black letters numbers most frequently called and "trouble" numbers—police, hospital, emergency room and personal physician.

Aids to dialing include plastic collars with large black numerals on white, or vice versa, that fit around rotary dials. Some of these overlay dials have raised numerals. For standard push-button phones there are self-adhesive large numbers that can be peeled off a sheet and pasted over the phone buttons. Then there are special phones with jumbo push buttons and oversized numerals for home and office.

More expensive are the high-tech memory phones that can be programmed to store and retrieve frequently called and emergency numbers. The push of one button dials the whole number. Partially sighted and blind owners of these phones rate them as one of their most useful, efficient aids.

Security

It used to be that only the rich worried about burglars, but now anyone with a TV set is a likely victim. According to police, the handicapped are favorite targets for burglars. A police officer told me, "Most burglars these days are lazy young criminals who are always on the lookout for easy jobs and victims who aren't likely to put up resistance. The elderly and people with handicaps like poor sight are singled out."

The partially sighted, often unable to recognize people at a distance on the street, are unlikely to spot suspicious behavior in strangers loitering in the neighborhood or prowling apartment house corridors.

Recognizing the vulnerability of the elderly and the handicapped, many police departments have issued special instructions for their self-protection. Maryland's Prince Georges County Police Department with the county's Office for Coordination of Services to the Handicapped has published the pamphlet, *Crime Prevention Tips for the Disabled.*

The pamphlet's Home Security section gives these tips:

- Never open your door to a stranger. Always verify the identity and purpose of the individual before opening the door.
- Avoid having a salesperson into your home, unless a friend or relative is present with you.
- Never let a stranger calling by phone know you are alone or that you are disabled.
- Plan an avenue of escape from each room in your residence for use in case of an emergency, such as a break-in or a disaster.
- Make sure you have proper locks on doors and windows —and use them—when you are at home, as well as when you go out.

Sergeant Robert Gross of the District of Columbia's Community Relations Unit adds this advice for home security:

- Dead bolt locks should be on all doors that have access from the outside. (Burglars have little trouble opening ordinary door locks with plastic credit cards.)
- To secure windows, especially on the first floor, drill a hole through both window frames and insert a bolt. Sliding glass doors should be secured in the same way or with a sturdy broom handle braced against the door frame.
- Shrubbery should be cut to waist-high level and should never cover windows.

As crime has increased in suburban and rural areas, more home owners who live alone or feel they are likely targets for intruders are installing electronic alarm systems, the ensuing peace of mind more than justifying the expense. Years ago, when I spent my summer vacations with a friend who lives in a coastal Maine town, we never locked the doors when we went out. Recently, as her sight diminished and a rash of burglaries occurred in the area, she had an elaborate electronic alarm system installed. Now, like millions of other Americans, every time she leaves the house, she not only locks the doors and windows but sets the alarm system.

Officers in police department community relations units, as part of their crime prevention duties, advise individuals about security measures for their homes and are especially helpful to people with handicaps. These officers not only advise residents individually, but give talks at meetings of community groups, including self-help groups of the partially sighted, who, to the ever watchful and calculating criminal, are targets for intruders and attackers.

In summary, adapting the personal environment to enhance its visibility need not involve drastic, expensive changes; much can be achieved by applying principles of effective lighting, sensible furniture arrangement, ingenious use of color, texture and contrast, and eliminating hazards that, unnoticed as sight declines, have transformed the familiar, safe haven into a danger zone.

Some hard-nosed decisions may be necessary in the process of adapting the home to new visual requirements. A favorite, bulky armchair or oversize table may have to be discarded to reduce "country-house clutter" and open up rooms for easy, safe passage.

Assessing the arrangement of one's household possessions can be accomplished with adaptational planning for a different pattern of living, a positive experience that has made some people with poor vision wonder how they had put up with things as they were.

7

Coping with Low Vision

How one copes with low vision is as personal as one's name. There are plenty of guidelines and much psychological advice, but how those guidelines will be used and the psychological advice followed depend on each individual. In this era of conformity, the partially sighted display a refreshing individuality in their patterns of coping with low vision.

I have yet to meet a partially sighted person who, after being told he or she had a serious eye defect that could lead to blindness, sat down and worked out a strategy for dealing with it. What usually happens is that they improvise their lives as they go along, at first hoping that the prognosis isn't true and then, as sight declines, accommodating to it, getting stronger glasses, buying hand magnifiers, but not accepting the fact of failing vision. When at a certain point self-deception is no longer possible, when the reality is all too evident, some will seek help from eye doctors, often the first step to a low vision clinic. Others will cover their visual defect by various ruses. Still others may begin a gradual retreat from social life and careers.

Strongly influencing how a person will adapt to declining sight is how an eye doctor presents the diagnosis and explains the nature of the impairment and its likely course. Though a doctor informs a patient of the situation with great finesse and consideration—not bludgeoning the patient with "You're going blind"—the doctor's words and voice may be drowned out by the patient's "internal noise" set off by fear and agitation. The patient will need a private time to contemplate a future suddenly quite different from the one planned on. On a subsequent visit to the eye doctor, the patient will be more thoughtful, better able to ask questions and to understand what the doctor says about the visual defect, its probable course, possible medical treatment, and types of visual aids that could enhance vision as it declines or, as may be the case, stabilizes.

For people with questing minds, a first step in the coping strategy is to learn about their eye disorder. Dorothy Stiefel, of Corpus Christi, Texas, after learning she had retinitis pigmentosa, experienced an emotional nightmare, tormented by fear, anger, self-pity and depression. As she relates in her booklet *Dealing with the Threat of Loss,* "My hurting would conjure up spurts of passion I couldn't believe I possessed . . . I had no way to work out my inner trauma . . . I was alone."

She became a student of retinitis pigmentosa, learning about the nature of the disorder and its vagaries. "I spent countless hours in medical libraries trying to sort out the technical language. I carried a dictionary wherever I went in search of articles written about retinitis pigmentosa." As she began to recognize what the symptoms of "night blindness" and "tunnel vision" meant, she became less intimidated by her vision problems. "It's the unknowable and the wretched things that tear you up. Each time I gained a little more insight, I became that less fearful." Armed with newly acquired knowledge, Mrs. Stiefel felt for the first time "in control again, equipped with enough ammunition to ward off insanity, and with awareness skills to cope with my visual limitations."

With the resurgence of control and self-confidence, she was able to reach out to others going through similar experiences. "Out of all the pain, fear, doubt, guilt, and self-depreciation came a renewed person," she writes. This renewed person organized and directed the Texas Association of Retinitis Pigmentosa, published regular newsletters, wrote articles about retinitis pigmentosa and the emotional aspects of sight loss, and a series of booklets. Not content with this new career as a journalist, Mrs. Stiefel started another career, managing a successful floral-arrangement business.

Among the many influences on how a person copes with severe sight loss—whether sudden or that point in declining vision when glasses no longer help—is the stage in the life span when that crisis occurs. It's not so much chronological age that matters in this situation, but where the person is in the developmental spectrum, whether the person is still striving toward goals or has settled into a purposeless routine.

Children with partial sight are mainstreamed these days from the outset of their school experience. Most of them, strongly supported by teachers and special educators, survive what Dr. Colenbrander calls the "crucible of peer rejection," though some, unable to endure ridicule and taunts, respond with angry defiance, refuse to use bizarre-looking optical aids and may even drop out of school.

Sometimes blunt talk may be more effective with hypersensitive teenagers than sympathetic reasoning. Richard Bignell, headmaster of the John Aird's School for the Partially Sighted, in London, tells about a fifteen-year-old girl who visited the school about the time she was preparing for "O" level examinations. Her vision was very poor, and though she had excellent low vision aids prescribed by a hospital, she refused to use them for fear of being embarrassed in the classroom. Mr. Bignell said to the girl, "Now this is absolutely stupid. Why worry about what the other girls say when almost certainly in a few years' time you won't know them? Yet because of your worries about the feelings of your classmates you are putting at risk your vital 'O' level examinations which could well dictate your career for the rest of your life. What you have to do, like all visually handicapped people, is to fight for yourself and look after number one. Think about yourself and your own needs rather than worry about other people's attitudes and feelings." Soon after getting that advice, the girl wrote to Mr. Bignell that she had started to use her visual aids in class. What she found out was that her classmates didn't make fun of her, but, when it was obvious from the aids that she had a visual handicap, her classmates wanted to help her.

Dr. Economon, who treats many partially sighted young people in her ophthalmological practice in Washington, D.C., says, "Young people find that they can see well enough for jobs or school work using regular glasses. They 'accommodate' to avoid using conspicuous low vision aids and some of these young people become quite skillful in concealing their eye defects. Some use their aids in secret, but never on dates. Older people who can't get along without their low vision aids are apt to be less self-conscious about using them."

Rarely do partially sighted young people talk about their fears and humiliations except, perhaps, to a trusted counselor. But they can reveal their inner suffering wordlessly as I observed in the corridor of an eye clinic. The corridor was lined with empty plastic chairs, except for one occupied by a boy, about sixteen years old, his thin, angular body slumped motionless, his head hanging down almost to his chest. I couldn't see his eyes; they were concealed by the long visor of the baseball cap pulled over his ears. In his posture and unnatural stillness, the boy portrayed the loneliness and unhappiness that so many partially sighted adults express in words.

Sudden sight loss at any age from car crashes, physical violence, retinal detachment or other causes is a catastrophe to which few can adjust without help from psychotherapists, no matter how supportive family and friends may be. Shock and grief are followed by a period of mourning. This mourning was not only approved by workers with the blind, but encouraged as a necessary stage in the process of adjusting to blindness. Underlying that concept of blindness was the conviction that loss of sight was as irrevocable as death. As recently as two decades ago, those who worked with the blind stated as a requisite for rehabilitation services that the blind abandon all hope of sight recovery and accept the "death of the eyes." Today surgical and other medical treatment have changed that attitude. By restoring some vision for hundreds of thousands, it legitimizes hope as a factor in coping with sight loss, especially among the young, who will benefit from research already well advanced in laboratories.

Gradual decline of sight, though frightening, at least allows time for adjustment and, in many cases, preparation for planning new careers, changing priorities, and adapting homes for safe and convenient living.

Though much is being done to enhance poor vision in the elderly, they encounter special psychological and emotional impediments to adapting to reduced sight. Dr. Alfred A. Rosenbloom, former president of the Illinois College of Optometry, in Chicago, told me,

"Elderly people are apt to accept loss of vision as an inevitable result of aging, and consequently many of them don't ask for help. Many who do seek help can't articulate their needs as effectively as younger people, which can make it difficult for practitioners to help them. And some elderly people don't cooperate in the treatment for fear that, if their sight is improved markedly, they will lose disability benefits. Others lose interest in a treatment program when they find out it doesn't restore their former good vision, which is really what they want. Improving the vision they have is not enough."

Studies of why some elderly people don't seek help for their visual problems cite a reluctance to reveal their age and income, transportation problems, and lack of physical endurance. Many older people shun rehabilitation centers for the blind that also serve the partially sighted, for fear of being labeled blind. Though shutting themselves off from organized sources of help, most partially sighted elderly people develop ways of adapting to their visual limitations that enable them to function in a sighted world.

Among the visually impaired with whom he has worked as a volunteer, James G. Chandler says the one word that best epitomizes their strongest motivation is *survival.*

> They have to get through each day solving one problem after another. Preparing meals may not seem a great problem to the rest of us, but if you put yourself in the

place of someone who can barely see, you can imagine how taxing it is to find ingredients, put them together, set the oven to the right temperature or light a burner. How do they find what they want in stores, especially these days when so many stores are self-service? How does a timid old lady find out where the rest rooms are? It's no wonder so many elderly people with poor sight huddle at home, don't go out, afraid of encounters, and brusk "Why don't you look where you're going?" But they have to take a first step, put the toe in the water as it were, test the world and venture into it.

Sometimes unforeseen events force older people out of their psychological cocoons. Often a rediscovery of will occurs when they lose in one way or another someone they had depended on. An elderly near-blind woman who had coped very well for forty years because her devoted husband had waited on her hand and foot was suddenly widowed. Almost helpless, faced with entering a nursing home, she went to an eye doctor who told her she had cataracts. At seventy-four, she had the cataracts removed and regained her sight and her self-confidence to the extent of making regular plane trips from Florida to Boston to visit her daughter and grandchildren.

In his consumer guide to low vision, *Eye Trumpets,* published by the Low Vision Association of Ontario, Canada, Bill Carroll says a serious problem for some low visioned people

> is a kind of paralysis of action which results from the fact their vision is *diminishing.* They worry about spending

money on an aid that may work well now but be useless to them in a year or two. They worry about becoming helpless.

The publishers of *Eye Trumpets* believe we should all use the vision we've got while we've got it.

Too much worry about the vision we won't have in five or ten years can keep us from making the best use of the vision we do have right now.

Our persistent advice to people with diminishing vision is that they proceed as though their vision wasn't diminishing—that they do everything possible to get the maximum benefits from whatever level of vision they have. If that means buying a particular low vision aid now, we say buy it. . . . The experience you gain using a less powerful vision aid now will serve you well in using a more powerful one later on.

Mimi Winer lost her sight to a rare retinal disorder while only in her early thirties. But together with another woman she founded the first self-help group for the partially sighted in Boston. Once a month they met to talk about their eye problems and to share their feelings, their fears, anger, sense of isolation, emotions most of them could not express to family and friends.

"It was a healing process," Mrs. Winer said in an interview. "By helping each other, we helped ourselves. We were constantly making adjustments to changes in vision, every day or few weeks another problem. As word spread about our group, others joined us. Though we consulted professionals, we ran our own show instead of having professionals take charge. In the beginning, professionals resented us. They thought we were moving into their territory, but we convinced them that ours was a kind of mutual support none of us could find anywhere else."

When the group, which met alternately in various members' homes, became too large for an exchange of the warm, personal feelings they needed, Mrs. Winer organized smaller groups of six to ten. "Between meetings we kept in touch with each other by regular 'buddy' phone calls just to chat as friends do or to help each other get through one of those bad spells that those whose sight is failing experience. Group members with fairly good residual vision gathered information about low vision clinics and aids, talking books, and publications for the partially sighted. Almost totally blind members demonstrated daily living techniques to those facing eventual sight loss." Mrs. Winer established the Vision Foundation, a national resource for information about low vision now situated in Watertown, Massachusetts.

Adjusting to a New Self-image

According to psychologists, we have a subconscious "fixed age" that remains constant, no matter how old we become. No one knows exactly how we select that secret age, but if you ask people what their fixed age is, they can generally tell you after only a moment's reflection. Most commonly they set that age from about eighteen to twenty-five years. This fixed age is tied up in some way with the self-image, that amalgam of impressions about ourselves, our appearance, intelligence and personality.

Severe visual impairment assaults that self-image, forcing us to construct a new one. The man of fifty-three whose fixed age is twenty-one and whose self-image is that of the football hero he once was is hard put to reconcile that vigorous athlete and "big man on campus" with the hesitant, anxiety-ridden half-blind man he has become. Acknowledging the discrepancy is the first tentative step toward dealing realistically with the visual handicap, a private, internal struggle that doesn't show up on any charts. But by gradually, though reluctantly, modifying the cherished self-image to bring it more in line with the new one that others see, he is rewarded by a sense of control, of being in charge of his own body as he once was as an athlete.

Irreversible loss of some sight does not change a person's character, it merely modifies the personality to some degree, according to the Reverend Thomas J. Carroll, who says in his book *Blindness* that the condition does not give the visually handicapped a new personality structure, but merely emphasizes the one they brought to the condition. Though no new personality structure is set up, "the old one becomes more set than ever in its basic channels . . . Currents that have long flowed underneath may come flooding to the surface."

Adapting to a less flattering self-image and a new self-identity is a test of resolution and strength of will that account in part for the differences in how two people with the same eye disorder react to it. Bill Berger, the New York literary agent mentioned in a previous chapter, despite declining vision not only kept up his literary agency, but expanded it. By contrast, a

New York advertising copywriter about Berger's age, whose sight also was failing because of retinitis pigmentosa, gave up his job, left New York, and went to live with his mother in a small town. When I met him at a party, he was carrying the long flexible white cane, symbol of blindness. He talked quite freely about his retinal disease. While I was telling him about electronic aids being used by many people with retinitis pigmentosa, aids he had not heard about, I became aware of his mother standing beside him, fixing me with tight-lipped disapproval. Taking her son's arm, saying they must meet other guests, she led her blind "boy" away. How blind was he? Chances are he would never find out so long as his protective mother lived. He had retreated from the competitive world to a maternal sanctuary, reconstructing a new self-image, that of an attention-getting blind man.

Declining sight obliges a person to do some self-assessing based on where the person is in the life span, way of life, work, goals and plans. As a partially sighted man said to me, "You may have to turn your life around, sort things out, decide what's more important and adjust to new priorities. Sometimes they're old goals in different guises." The painter Degas as his sight declined switched to sculpture. Engineers have become computer programmers within their field of expertise. An insurance agent whose poor sight disqualified him for a driver's license, decided he wanted a college degree—and got it. A characteristic of coping with low vision is that as sight declines, even imperceptibly, self-reassessment goes on, often subconsciously, as choices are made in the process of adapting.

Many people with severe visual impairments have learned to function so well in business, restaurants and classrooms that others may be unaware of the handicap. Though I had attended several meetings at which she had presided, I didn't realize Mrs. B. was nearly blind until we lunched together for the first time. An administrator in a national agency, she is a handsome woman in her forties, always stylishly dressed, poised, articulate. Her animated face and beautiful eyes give no hint of a visual disorder, but at that first lunch she surprised me by taking from her handbag a small standing magnifier through which she scanned the menu held close to her eyes. She compounded my surprise by telling me she could not distinguish my features across the table. Yet she travels alone throughout the country, conducts meetings, serves as consultant to other agencies, and skis.

Macular degeneration, the cause of her visual problem, manifested itself when Mrs. B. was in her teens. Its progress was slow, and during the early period of sight deterioration, she married and had a child. The eventual breakup of the marriage she attributes in part to her sight loss. Though her husband was proud of her success as a business woman, he couldn't cope with being married to a "flawed" woman, as she put it.

"When a partner can't accept a flaw, in my case the loss of most of my vision," she told me, "there's bound to be deep-seated resentment in a spouse over having to adjust to it. Of course, the situation in a marriage can be almost as bad if a husband or wife is overly solicitous and so helpful the visually impaired spouse feels inadequate and may become overdependent. There's a fine line between giving too much help and not being supportive enough. And this is true in relations with one's children. I've learned that the best system for keeping family relations harmonious is to learn to do as much as possible myself, doing small chores and errands and limiting my requests for help to the big things I can't possibly do myself, like driving the car."

How successfully people with partial sight will cope with their many challenges is usually unpredictable; as yet there is no way to measure the resilience of the human spirit. After surgery had restored some sight to one eye—a retinal detachment had totally destroyed the sight in the other eye—Robert Greenhalgh applied for a job with a British rehabilitation agency and was told he was unqualified because of his defective vision. Ten years later Mr. Greenhalgh headed that rehabilitation service in which he had been denied a job. Nor had his ophthalmologist encouraged him to seek professional work, but as chairman of Britain's Partially Sighted Society he not only administers its many programs, but is a consultant and lecturer on low vision.

"Ophthalmologists should not make social judgments," he told me. "In the first place they do not know what useful vision is and too often underestimate a patient's ability to adjust. It's hard for anyone, not only ophthalmologists, to predict, because of the many variables in partial sight. It's not necessary to see everything any more than it's necessary to hear everything. The mind screens out an enormous amount of visual information and allows only a small quantity through the net. How well a person uses what sight he or she has depends on social and educational background, what the person has been encouraged and trained to see, experience, focus of education, and ability to guess."

Sighted people receive more visual information than they need for functioning competently, but, Mr. Greenhalgh said, people with low vision do not have this luxury, but must make the most of a very limited amount of information. "Because the quantity of information is reduced and a vast array of incidental visual information is absent, I have to work hard at interpreting what I'm seeing."

To aid him in interpretation, Mr. Greenhalgh has developed what he calls the "dim's drill." He starts out by checking his scanning to make sure he's using his maximum visual field. He assesses the lighting to find out if it affects his depth perception as well as his color vision. He focuses far to near and back again. He looks carefully around a room to get some idea of the layout and identifies significant points—doorways, chairs and tables. "I get myself fully alert, so that my reactions are fast, and make sure my muscles are up to scratch. To test my mental alertness, I sometimes do a couple of quick mental arithmetic problems." He is ready for his encounter with the sighted world.

I had occasion to observe Mr. Greenhalgh's "dim's

drill" in London when he escorted me from his office to a nearby restaurant, ordered our lunch, and later took me to the tube (subway) station, got on the train with me and saw to it that I got off at the right stop, an impressive demonstration by a man, secure in a sense of himself despite severely limited vision, using it with maximum efficiency.

Psychological "swings," familiar to everyone, are exacerbated in the visually impaired by constant frustration—being unable to do easily and quickly what once was done effortlessly, frustrations that bring on upsurges of feelings of inadequacy and self-pity, even rage, and sheer physical and emotional fatigue brought on by the ceaseless effort of trying to fit in and live like sighted people in a vision-oriented world.

Making matters worse are fluctuations in vision common to the partially sighted. Inexplicably, they see better some days than on others. Apart from the unsettling effects on the partially sighted themselves, often raising false hopes of miraculous cures, these fluctuations are confusing to family members and friends, some of whom suspect the partially sighted person is faking poor vision on his or her "bad" days, a visual variation on the old saying, "None so deaf as those who will not hear."

In *Eye Trumpets,* Bill Carroll writes:

> Some low visioned people feel constantly off balance because their level of vision *fluctuates,* or seems to fluctuate, from one situation to another or day to day.

> Vision fluctuation is a serious nuisance for all of us which can sometimes be minimized by things like adjusting the level or range of light or switching from one low vision aid to another. Sometimes we can do little more than tolerate it.
>
> Such fluctuations can make performing visual tasks more difficult. They rarely make visual performance impossible.

Though most of these fluctuations cannot be explained medically (in diabetics, the cause is attributed to changes in blood-sugar levels), people who experience these changes in acuity have explanations of their own, weather conditions for one. Some people with macular degeneration say they see better on overcast days. A man with retinitis pigmentosa told me that contrary to the usual pattern of that disease, his vision is better at night than in daylight.

Stress undoubtedly is a factor in vision fluctuation. Dorothy Stiefel found in the early stages of retinitis pigmentosa that fear of "failing" caused nausea, and as her stomach knotted, her nerves tensed, and as she "froze," she writes in her booklet, "I actually blocked my vision psychologically. I saw less at the terrible times because I had worked myself into an emotional frenzy." Later after mobility and orientation training, she rediscovered the fun of sports and in taking brisk walks in the familiar neighborhood. As she regained a sense of control, power and security, her tension attacks diminished, and though her sight continued to decline, it did so less erratically.

Social Relations

Among the reasons many people with defective vision try to cover up is fear of losing their jobs, of being labeled blind if they take rehabilitation courses, and especially of being rejected by the opposite sex. Dating is a major concern of partially sighted young adults and of older singles as well. In some self-help groups, dating is a popular topic of discussion. How do you meet people? Should you admit you have a vision problem if they haven't already noticed? One young man in a self-help group told about going on a first date carrying his white cane—the date ended at the front door. At a dance, a young woman whose sight was minimal approached a tall, slender man and asked him to dance. The tall man with close-cropped hair turned out to be a woman, very indignant at having been mistaken for a man. Some partially sighted people have replied to ads in the "Personals" sections of newspapers and magazines, and some have used computer dating services.

Among the many anxieties besetting the partially sighted is fear of losing sexual drive and attraction. In psychiatric language, the eyes are an *erogenous zone,* organs of sexual excitation. Painters, poets and lovers have immortalized the attributes of the eyes, their beauty and power to arrest, haunt, invite, question, and transmit messages of desire, melancholy, hatred, adoration. Being unable to see the eyes of others deprives one of what has been called "the little consoling flirtations of everyday life."

In his book *Ordinary Daylight,* Andrew Potok says that not being able to see made him feel undesirable, unmanly, and he laments not being able to engage in the sophisticated language of the eyes, of having no access to the "eyes' ambiguities, no playful enigmatic dialogue, no sexual finesse. I felt particularly loutish without my eyes . . . I wondered what signs I was missing, whether her countenance was sparkling or dull, bored or preoccupied or aroused. I yearned for the absolute truth of the eyes' and the body's involuntary code."

In the course of being reassured about his sexuality, Potok discovered that the inhibitor he feared was not so much organic, but rather his obsessive preoccupation with his defective sight. As someone has put it, visual defects do not geld a man or spay a woman; confidence in one's sexual powers is the essential aphrodisiac.

Partially sighted women seem not so concerned about losing sexual power as of losing feminine allure. As one woman told me, though a woman may not be able to see very well, she can listen and show her interest by facial expression and animation. A partially sighted man I asked for clues to whether or not a woman was attractive said he could tell by the way she talked, the sound of her voice, her perfume and hair style, and the way she joked and laughed. "One clue used to be body contact in dancing," he said, "but today's style of dancing doesn't give much opportunity for that. Disco dancing, couples separated, doing their own thing, deprived us of a pretty reliable clue to physical attraction."

Among the partially sighted there's no consensus about the chances of successful marriage in which both partners have severe visual impairments. A businessman, almost blind from birth, says his successful career would have been impossible without his sighted wife, who managed the household, took care of their children, and in numerous ways compensated for his poor vision. Some partially sighted couples find that coping with common problems, giving each other psychological and emotional support, binds them together in a union often stronger than that between many sighted couples.

But when one partner begins to lose sight, a tremendous strain can be placed on a marriage, especially if the marriage is on shaky ground to begin with. Too often the bitter saying, "Loss of sight—loss of spouse," becomes a reality. Unfair as it may seem, much of the burden for making a marriage survive this stressful situation falls on the partner whose sight is failing. It's during this distressing period of readjustment that low vision clinics and self-help groups can provide practical aids, optical and psychological, that enable the partially sighted spouse to sustain the relationship and save the marriage.

Etiquette Tips for the Sighted

The visually impaired themselves offer suggestions to those who wish to be helpful when it's obvious they need help in an unfamiliar or stressful situation. At the top of the list is: Don't force help, ask first if the person would like to be helped. Even the most self-reliant partially sighted people get into baffling situations. For example, when the familiar sidewalk they walk along everyday is being repaired and is blocked by barriers that a person with low vision can see only vaguely. Be precise when giving directions—"Left" or "Right" or "Straight ahead," but not "Over there." In groups, avoid using the personal pronoun *he* or *she* when referring to someone in the group. Identify the person by name. It's not enough to say, "Here's a flight of steps." Specify whether the steps go up or down. On social occasions always identify yourself when you approach a partially sighted person. And don't be offended if a person who can barely see doesn't shake your hand when you hold it out. Take his or her hand and shake it. When you leave, say you're leaving. People with low vision complain that they find they're talking to themselves after someone has made an unobtrusive departure at a cocktail party where unobtrusive leave-taking is part of the circulation ritual.

Resources

The best resource for help in dealing with defective vision is private and internal—the individual's determination, intelligence, adaptability and, in large measure, courage.

Robert E. Brown has been in a race against blindness for thirty years. As a young man he was told he had a rare, incurable retinal disease that would eventually blind him. Despite the grim prognosis, he married, fathered four children, and worked for many years in the federal government as an employment counselor and personnel administrator. When his sight became so bad he could not function adequately on the job, he gave it up and discovered computers as a means of "keeping ahead of blindness." With technical advice from computer experts, he devised a system that enables him to continue his career as an employment counselor, assisting veterans and others seeking jobs in government and private industry. Besides helping job hunters prepare résumés, he does free-lance editing on contract and, as a computer adviser, helps clients set up computer systems designed for their special needs.

When I interviewed him in his office, an attractively renovated basement apartment in a townhouse on Capitol Hill in Washington, D.C., he demonstrated his ingenious computer system, an Apple IIe linked up with a Vtek DP-10 on which he types in whatever size letters (as large as six inches) his visual acuity at the moment requires. His sight has deteriorated over the years to the point where only a tiny part of the retina is usable. Yet he continues to handle a full work load and to experiment with new electronic equipment, which enables him to "keep ahead of blindness." His latest acquisition is a five-pound portable computer ("Small Talk") with voice synthesizer, small screen and printer he uses for note taking at meetings, now that he can no longer see to write.

This hard-driving, innovative, almost blind man who for thirty years has been coping with declining sight says the technology is here for the partially sighted. "They should learn to use it instead of complaining about their poor vision. The blind traditionally have been encouraged to let others do things for them and to feel they are something special. It's easy for them to give up and play the role of recipients. What people with severe vision problems need is advice on the availability of new technology and training in its use."

Computers have become a family affair for the Browns—the elder son is a computer service technician and a daughter a computer science major at Maryland University.

People with low vision, formerly in a sort of limbo, neither blind nor sighted, now have a great number of resources for helping them cope successfully with their handicap. They have been "discovered" by private and public agencies, by rehabilitation specialists, manufacturers of optical and nonoptical visual aids, by eye-care doctors, and above all, they have discovered one another.

Heading the list of resources for helping the partially sighted cope with poor vision are, of course, low vision clinics, now in every major city throughout the United States. But unless an ophthalmologist or optometrist refers a patient to a low vision clinic, it's up to the patient to find one. Sources of information about low vision clinics include:

State and local medical societies.
Local associations of optometrists and ophthalmologists.
Colleges of optometry.
Ophthalmology departments in medical centers and hospitals.
State and local associations of rehabilitation professionals.
Local public health department rehabilitation services.
State Commissions for the Blind and partially sighted.
Local agencies serving the partially sighted.
Phone directory listings of low vision clinics and private practitioners specializing in low vision services.

Low vision self-help or support groups, on the increase throughout the country, generally attract members who have common interests and educational backgrounds. The membership of National Capital

Citizens with Low Vision (NCCLV) of Washington, D.C., a consumer, advocacy and self-help organization, is made up largely of business men and women, lawyers, teachers and secretaries interested in social events, and sports, including skiing and hiking—one member is an experienced mountain climber. The group is formally structured, with bylaws and elected officers, and issues a monthly newsletter. Regular monthly meetings feature discussions of getting about the city using public transportation, special services for the visually impaired, legal rights on the job, and problems in coping with everyday situations. Copies of the NCCLV leaflet "We Take a Closer Look," describing the organization's activities are sent to ophthalmologists and optometrists in the Washington area. Low vision specialists are invited to talk about the latest developments in optical and electronic aids, and medical advances in treating eye disorders. Though a professional therapist might not consider the meetings as group therapy, they definitely have a therapeutic effect through sharing experiences and in the comfort of being with people who encounter similar problems in a world geared to the sighted. As one member said to me, "Being with others who have similar frustrations and tensions and who realize how much energy it takes to function in business surrounded by sighted people, I don't feel I have to stand at attention all the time. At our meetings, we relax and even laugh together about some of our experiences."

In contrast to this structured group are the more

informal support groups under the aegis of Vision Foundation stemming from the original group that Mimi Winer organized. "These groups are all different," Mrs. Winer told me. "Each moves with the needs of the particular participants. Sometimes low vision devices are discussed, sometimes they're not. The pain of vision loss seems to be the biggest issue for new participants, while practical matters like aids and devices are more intriguing to veteran participants. Of course, for the few participants who have lost all sight low vision is no longer an issue. Between meetings, members keep in touch through the 'buddy' system."

The base of these self-help groups, according to Mrs. Winer, is a nucleus of men and women who, besides having a common bond in vision problems, are congenial and able to give each other understanding support. In her guidelines for organizing a self-help-support network for people with declining sight, Mrs. Winer says, "Our self-help groups are formed when there are enough people in a local area to set them up. This method reduces major transportation expenses. We've found that eight to ten people in a self-help group works best. Each group is set up by one or two coordinators, who work with the host or hostess in making arrangements for the meetings, scheduling and transportation."

Occasionally, sighted members of a family also need "buddies." "When they request it," said Mrs. Winer, "we put them in touch with appropriate people. Our groups are open-ended and flexible. People come into them and go out as they need. Sometimes a sighted spouse attends a meeting. But no matter how understanding your family is and wants to be, there's no way they can understand the grief and anxieties that are part of your very private self, something deeper than worries about how you're going to cope with everyday demands. In our self-help groups the men and women understand, and we can talk about our private fears more openly with each other than with members of our own family."

According to Fran Weisse, manager of the Vision Foundation's Information Center, most young and middle-aged adults with low vision, bolstered by a wide choice of aids, optical and nonoptical, and by eye doctors and volunteer and public agencies, manage fairly well in coping with everyday demands. But, says Mrs. Weisse, there are times when personal situations overwhelm them beyond the capacity of the group to help them, and they need individual professional counseling. Most low vision clinics have psychotherapists or specially trained social workers on their staffs to help in these crisis situations. Some partially sighted people prefer to go to psychotherapists in private practice. When I asked a man going through a traumatic phase with the help of a therapist in private practice how he had selected his therapist, he said he had looked for someone who had experienced at some time in his life a trauma equivalent in degree to slowly going blind. The psychotherapist he selected had been a combat soldier in Vietnam.

Adaptability Training

Mobility, orientation and sensitivity training, originally developed for the blind, increasingly is being adapted to the needs of the partially sighted, who may see quite well in some situations, but not in others. It's possible, for instance, for some people to see quite well indoors where light is diffused, but to be blinded outdoors by bright sunlight.

Mobility training is geared to helping the visually impaired develop skills for getting about independently and safely. As sight diminishes, there's likely to come a time when a person begins to feel unsure about his or her ability to function as a pedestrian or user of public transportation. Numerous public and private agencies sponsor mobility training as part of rehabilitation programs, but their existence may be unknown to partially sighted people who could benefit from them. For one thing, many of these agencies, identified primarily with services for the blind, have not publicized services for the partially sighted. And their phone directory listings do not make it easy for those seeking vision rehabilitation services to find them. Some agencies have a means test. People whose incomes may be even slightly above the baseline of that test are not eligible for the training, the official attitude being that "if you aren't poor enough, we won't help you." As a result of this straitjacket on rehabilitation training, some enterprising mobility and orientation instructors have gone into private practice, training those who need and can afford their services.

Because mobility training was initially developed for the blind, some instructors advocate putting the partially sighted "under the blindfold" or sleep shades. Those who advocate simulating blindness do so on the theory that if blindness occurs, the person will be able to adapt more readily to it. Speaking as a partially sighted consumer, Richard Bignell, outspoken headmaster of a school for the partially sighted in London, criticizes the practice of using masklike devices in mobility training. "I think this practice is abominable, and I can see no justification at all for people with sight, however limited that sight may be, being plunged into a world of darkness and treated as if they are totally blind. Sight is the major sense and is incredibly important, though it might be severely impaired. How can people who are handicapped reach a peak of performance if their remaining sight is to be ignored?"

Theresa Travis, supervisor of rehabilitation at the Columbia Lighthouse for the Blind, when retinitis pigmentosa had severely reduced her vision, signed up for mobility training. The instructor looked at her high heels and told her she would have to get flat heel shoes. Mrs. Travis told the instructor that high heels were what she wore and that's what she would continue to wear. The instructor, defeated by this display of spunk, gave her mobility training as she walked with ease on high heels.

Orientation training, often combined with mobility

training, concentrates on outdoor environment, helping those with low vision to size up traffic and spot the location of buildings, doorways and stairs.

Sensitivity training helps increase the efficiency of senses other than sight—hearing, touch, smell and taste—to compensate for diminished sight. Many partially sighted whose other senses seem to be functioning in top form are skeptical about being able to improve them to any useful degree. But most, after some training, realize that they have been using their senses lackadaisically. One skeptical trainee, who could scarcely see, was given the assignment of opening a milk carton. If you can't see the printed instructions on the carton, how do you know which side to pry open? At first the trainee's fingers could sense no difference in the folds of the carton, but gradually, concentrating on her fingers, almost listening to their sensitivity, she detected the fold to be pried open. That success changed her attitude toward sensory enhancement and she went on to refine her other senses. As she became more skillful and self-reliant, she emerged from the psychological cocoon she had wrapped herself in, joined a self-help group, and helped others cope with eye defects like hers. She credits that milk carton with being the turning point in her adaptability training.

What George Bernard Shaw said about health applies equally to vision: Use it, "even to the point of wearing it out. That is what it is for." How you use it and how well you cope with its imperfection is a personal matter that depends on your determination, flexibility and expertise in using the resources now available.

Coping with New Vision

Humankind accommodates many oddities, among them are those whose sight has been restored and who do not consider it an unmitigated blessing. Surgeons have learned not to expect gratitude from every patient whose sight they have restored. A woman who had lost her sight from cataracts while in her early twenties, for forty-five years had visualized herself in her mind's eye as the pretty young woman whose image she had last seen in the mirror. After cataract surgery, when she looked in the mirror and saw a wrinkled, white-haired old lady she became hysterical and railed against the surgeon who had restored her sight, blaming him for the image in the mirror.

In his book, *The World Through Blunted Sight,* Patrick Trevor-Roper says:

> The least grateful patients are generally those whose cataracts have been removed and whose sight has been dramatically restored. They grumble endlessly at the inevitable but transient distortions caused by cataract spectacles. If they are old and have settled back into a comfortable dependence on others, it is upsetting to be told that they must fend for themselves again. A third of the blind in England are sightless because of a senile cataract that could well be removed, but they have some-

how failed to have recourse to this straightforward sight-saving operation, often, one suspects, because they cannot face the business of adjusting to a sighted world.

Trevor-Roper cites the case of a blind man who, at age fifty-two, had his sight restored by corneal grafts and found the world drab and full of such imperfections as flaking paint and who, as daylight faded, suffered from Hesperian depression, the universal evening melancholy that afflicts human beings and animals, a condition this formerly blind man had escaped when he could not see fading daylight.

> And, [writes Trevor-Roper] this cheerful, well-adjusted man, with a useful industrial job, who was happily reading braille in his spare time before the operation, became deeply disturbed thereafter and, losing his self-respect, soon died in unhappiness. The moral of this story should not be lightly overlooked.

For the newly sighted, the demands of learning to see are often overwhelming. Some whose sight has been restored must relate their previous sensing of objects, their size and shape, to what they see, a process that requires being taught not only about objects, but about such things as lines, curves, outlines, shadows and colors. In learning about the world around them, formerly vastly simplified by blindness, the memory is often taxed beyond its capacity by the myriad new objects encountered in the first few months of regained sight. Further complicating adjustment to sightedness is that rarely is restored sight perfect and to the confusion of the new visual world is added the task of learning to use special aids to enhance residual vision.

As cataract, corneal and retinal surgery restores some measure of sight to hundreds of thousands of Americans, it is time, as one low vision specialist says, to recognize the problems of this special category of partially sighted men, women and children—coping with new vision, reconciling newly acquired perceptions with imaginary images they have lived with during their sightlessness. Keeping afloat in the sighted world of which they have become part makes inordinate demands on the energy and intelligence, but according to the testimony of many whose sight has been even partially restored, once they get the knack of seeing, they feel not exactly "reborn," but "retuned" to the world and revitalized. Most are unfazed by such imperfections in the world as peeling paint.

8

Future Prospects

Estimates of the number of Americans whose impaired vision can't be improved by conventional eyewear range from two million to eleven million. But no one knows for sure.

Whatever the exact number of Americans with low vision—and no statistical net could have a fine enough mesh to catch all of them—it's safe to say there are millions. Though the incidence of total and near blindness is being reduced by optical surgery, new drugs, new methods of treating and preventing eye disorders, counterbalancing this reduction is the escalation of visual defects, mostly aging-related. But here again, other forces are at work.

It is as though the eyes in the last two decades have become a new physiological and social frontier attracting the attention of scientists, clinicians, rehabilitation and social workers, psychologists and industrialists. Agencies that heretofore served only the blind have begun branching out to provide services for the partially sighted.

The most dramatic developments have taken place in eye surgery. In 1978, eye surgeons were locked in debate over the risks of implanting a piece of plastic to replace the natural lens removed by cataract surgery. Eight years later, statistics revealed that of the one million cataract operations performed in 1985 in the United States, 85 percent involved the implantation of plastic lenses.

Leonardo da Vinci boiled a goat's eye to congeal the vitreous fluid so he could study that part of the eye. Until recently the prospect of surgically invading the vitreous brought shudders to ophthalmologists; the precious fluid, it was believed, would flow out and the eye would collapse. Now surgeons not only cut into the vitreous to remove invasive blood vessels, but, as the fluid is drawn out, they replace it with a synthetic substance. As surgical techniques are refined, the search goes on for improved substitutes for natural vitreous fluid.

Though lasers had been used for some years to seal rogue blood vessels characteristic of diabetic retinopathy, it was not until 1982 that lasers were designed specifically for treating retinal dysfunctions, glaucoma, and other eye disorders. When studies showed that laser treatment in the early stages of aging-related macular degeneration could halt its progress, eye surgeons added another instrument in combatting a disease that previously had been considered untreatable. Scientists developing medical applications for medical uses of lasers predict that the "magic beam of light" will have unlimited potential in treating eye disorders.

The breathtaking strides that eye surgery has made in just a decade are merely a portent of future progress. In the area of vision, the word *impossible* is being discredited by research, advances not only in treating eye disorders, but in other fields to which vision researchers are forging links, stimulated by the daring experiments of other scientists. Transplantation of organs and tissue fired the imaginations of optical scientists with the result that corneal transplants are now almost routine. Implantation of synthetic lenses after the removal of cataracts is now routine surgery in clinics. Torn and detached retinas are repaired with increasing success.

Where will vision researchers find their new frontier? Some predict it will be the retina, that fragile membrane, part of the brain, crucial to sight. Could healthy retinas be transplanted to replace diseased ones? At the University of Rochester (New York), Dr. Manuel del Cerro, professor of brain research, anatomy and ophthalmology, with his team of investigators, their work funded by the National Eye Institute, in 1985 announced their development of a new procedure for transplanting retinal tissue from rat embryos to adult rats. In some of the experiments, the scientists transplanted entire retinas and, for comparison purposes, transplanted "aggregates," tiny clusters of a few hundred or a thousand cells. The scientists sought to determine whether the transplanted tissue would take root and grow in the eye of the host rat and then perform the functions lost through damage to the host retina. Dr. Del Cerro predicts that if current and future research in the laboratory is successful, testing the transplantation of retinal tissue in human eyes may occur by the end of the 1980s.

Only a few decades ago even to speculate about regenerating optic nerves destroyed by degeneration or injury was considered sheer fantasy. When the optic nerve, the cable of nerves that transmits chemical signals from the retina to the visual centers of the brain, is destroyed, blindness results. Some hope for the regeneration of optic nerves stems from research at the Massachusetts Institute of Technology, where scientists have found a way of regenerating surgically severed sciatic nerves in rats. Professor Ioannis Yannas, director of these studies, announced in 1985 that for the first time regeneration occurred across gaps of nearly three quarters of an inch, using a chemical material that, acting as a sort of scaffold, guides tissue regrowth along natural lines, then disappears as regeneration takes place. This extraordinary advance will have application for repairing nerves damaged by accidents and disease and may eventually restore optic nerves.

At the Eye Research Institute of Retina Foundation in Boston, Drs. Max Snodderly and Peter Hartline in

1983 launched a research program to study ways of restoring sight. The program takes a nonsurgical approach, attacking the restoration of sight at a basic level. Building their studies on developments in neurological research, the two scientists are studying the way the brain combines information from the eyes with information from other senses, such as touch and hearing. According to the coinvestigators, if they can discover how the brain normally combines other senses with visual processing in the brain, they may learn how touch and hearing could be used to restore some visual function to blind or near-blind people.

In their initial studies, the two scientists have explored ways the nonvisual senses are combined with vision in mice and lower animals. Besides the senses (sight, sound, smell, taste and touch) common to human beings, they have explored in rattlesnakes a "sixth sense," an ability to sense heat radiation from warm-blooded prey, a sense evolved from the sense of touch or warmth on the skin. The investigators have found that the infrared sense in rattlesnakes forms in the brain a map of the space around the snake's head. In the same part of the brain, eyes also create a visual map. By interconnections between the two maps, many nerve cells "see" the same region of the world, both through the eyes and the infrared sense organs. Those nerve cells and the two maps account for the ability of snakes to locate and catch prey without "seeing" it. Snodderly and Hartline are trying to find out how snakes substitute another sense for sight.

Along with their studies of visual maps in the brain,

the two scientists are investigating how eye movements affect visual images. "We expect that visual aids that take advantage of the intrinsic organization of the brain to incorporate the influence of eye movements will be more effective and easier to use than visual aids now available," the coinvestigators predict.

At the Wilmer Eye Institute Laboratory of Physiological Optics of Johns Hopkins University School of Medicine, four major vision-related research projects were under way in 1985:

Studies of diseases such as diabetes that cause abnormal blood-vessel growth in the retina and criteria for identifying patients likely to develop those abnormal blood vessels in order to start treatment early enough to prevent the formation of those abnormalities.

Because 50 percent of the optic nerve must be damaged before conventional vision tests can detect any damage, Wilmer Eye Institute researchers are developing diagnostic criteria for detecting early optic-nerve damage, sometimes caused by abnormally high eye pressure from glaucoma.

Aging-related macular degeneration, the leading cause of impaired vision in Americans over sixty years of age, is a major focus of studies at Wilmer Eye Institute. Researchers are not only studying retinal functional and structural changes that occur in this degenerative disease, but are developing ways of identifying patients at high risk who would be candidates for early treatment.

Retinitis pigmentosa is also under intensive study at

the Wilmer Eye Institute. Toward the end of 1985, investigators began studies of visual performance by patients with impaired vision as a basis for classifying patients for vision rehabilitation.

These examples merely hint at the activity in vision research. Years after this book has been published you may read in your newspaper or hear on radio or television an announcement of the first implantation of retinal tissue in a human patient, or the first successful regeneration of an optic nerve, or a revolutionary way of restoring sight. These announcements will be the culmination of years of meticulous effort, false starts, persistence, applied imagination, and team work.

Developments in controlling or curing systemic diseases that adversely affect vision are reported with increasing frequency in journals and at medical meetings. In the forefront of such diseases is diabetes, affecting some ten million Americans. Insulin is the drug that keeps the disease under control, but administering the drug daily by injection is a serious problem for elderly people who can barely see to fill a syringe and inject the medicine. Scientists working on alternatives to injections reported in 1985 a new way of administering insulin—in a nasal spray. Early tests indicate the possible success of this method, but proof of its efficacy and safety will have to wait for extensive testing by clinicians. But for diabetics with low vision, this method would be a boon.

To discover whether eye problems and nerve damage resulting from diabetes can be prevented or slowed, the

National Eye Institute in collaboration with the pharmaceutical company Pfizer, Inc., launched a nationwide trial of a new drug, Sobinil, in 1985. The Sobinil Retinopathy Trial is the latest in a series of clinical trials sponsored by the National Eye Institute to evaluate various means of preventing and treating diabetic retinopathy, the leading cause of new cases of blindness each year in the United States.

Problems of administering daily medication plague not only diabetics, but also those who have glaucoma and must administer eyedrops as often as twenty-eight times a week. Many elderly people because of hand tremors or other disabilities cannot put drops in their eyes. Their dependence on others for this task, besides being an annoyance for everyone involved, further erodes independence and self-reliance. Researchers have devised an ocular insert similar to a contact lens. Called the Ocusert System, the device releases glaucoma medication in steady, controlled dosages continuously for seven days.

Ophthalmic pharmacology is now an integral part of eye research. Vision pharmacologists at centers throughout the country are developing and testing drugs for treating eye diseases. In 1984, the Eye Institute of Retina Foundation established its Ophthalmic Pharmacology Unit as part of its research team. Originally part of the Institute's laboratory for glaucoma pharmacology, its investigations were expanded to include a search for drugs for treating corneal diseases and some retinal disorders. In their new approach to treating retinal disease with drugs, members of the pharmacology unit are confident that drug therapy could alter the course of diabetic retinopathy and other retinal disorders characterized by leaking blood vessels or altered blood flow. Investigators in the unit are also exploring the conditions that result in abnormal cell growth in the retina following surgical repair of detached retinas. Drug therapy to prevent proliferation of cells could reduce the number of disheartening failures that occur after retinas have been reattached.

Keeping pace with the search for improved ways of controlling, curing or, better yet, preventing eye disorders, providing investigators, surgeons and low vision specialists with the tools are the biomedical engineers. In some instances, they produce instruments "on demand" for a particular procedure such as the "upside down" operating table for retinal surgery and tiny surgical instruments. But usually in eye-care centers and industrial plants, biomedical engineers are designing high-tech instruments for diagnosing eye disorders, treating them and assessing visual acuities. To a marked degree, future progress in biomedical engineering is expected in instruments for detecting in infants and young children early signs of disorders that can be corrected so that permanent damage to sight can be prevented. *Prevention* is a word you will be hearing more often in the late 1980s and beyond as these programs are stepped up.

Eye-care professionals in clinics and agencies are taking a more active part in prevention programs, and indications are that this trend will accelerate. Nationally, the American Academy of Ophthalmology, the American Optometric Association, and the Opticians Association of America, already engaged in public education programs about eye care, are expected to expand their efforts. Augmenting the public information programs of these professional groups, are the vision educational materials published and circulated by the National Eye Institute, the American Foundation for the Blind, and hundreds of local groups concerned about vision. A formidable ally in this public education process is the eye-care industry and producers of high-tech visual aids who, in the course of promoting their products, do a first-rate job of educating the public about impaired vision and what can be done about it.

Important improvements in rehabilitation and mobility research are being made by Drs. Steven J. LaGrow and Paul E. Ponchillia of Western Michigan University Department of Blind Rehabilitation and Mobility. In 1985, these two faculty members prepared a landmark report, an overview of visual impairment in the United States, predicted the impact of medical and optical techniques on sight loss by the year 2005, and gave a blueprint of the drastic changes rehabilitation services must make to meet the new demands and adapt to changes.

Dr. Ponchillia had entered Western Michigan University's Blind Rehabilitation and Mobility program as a recipient of its training following a tragic hunting accident in which his companion accidentally shot him full in the face, blinding him. Up to then, Dr. Ponchillia had spent his working days peering into a microscope, studying plant disease organisms, work that required keen eyesight. Following the accident, Dr. Ponchillia went through what is a classic pattern: rage, despair, hope, denial of his blindness, even the breakup of his marriage. At his work place, this scientist was given well-intentioned but humiliating tasks, such as answering the telephone.

Finally, accepting that he was irrevocably blind, he entered the rehabilitation program at Western Michigan University, realized that his research background, his own harrowing personal experience, and a strong desire to help others cope qualified him to seek a second career in rehabilitation training. He applied research methodology to developing innovations for coping with sight loss.

While training future rehabilitation instructors for service in the near future, Dr. Ponchillia and his colleague, Dr. LaGrow, looked ahead to the year 2005 and projected changes that will be required for rehabilitation services to meet the new demands of the visually impaired. They predict in their report that medical and optical techniques, and preventive programs will vastly reduce new cases of blindness in the United States. The dramatic changes ahead not only will affect millions of Americans who have defective vision, but will revolutionize eye care and rehabilitative services.

According to Drs. LaGrow and Ponchillia, the new type of rehabilitation specialist must be skilled in the use of electronics, able to develop training courses that use electronic media in local public and private agencies and provide educational services and training courses for other disciplines that provide health and social services to the visually impaired. With greater emphasis on preventing visual disorders, future training programs for students in rehabilitation should incorporate training in screening and detection procedures. These future rehabilitation practitioners will be trained for supervisory roles and for serving as consultants. Computer technology will become an integral part of the rehabilitation curriculum, incorporating research on its application as a teaching device as well as its uses as a tool for the visually impaired. Future rehabilitation training will place greater emphasis on low vision services, including preparing trainees to conduct research in low vision services aimed at developing instructional innovations to go hand in hand with medical and optical advances.

Developments in designs of optical aids will be more closely related to new types of vision assessment which pinpoint, for instance, usable areas of the retina. To help patients afflicted with macular degeneration, optical scientists are expected to develop aids that enhance the area of peripheral vision used as a substitute for damaged central vision. Though contact lenses are considered conventional eyewear these days, in many instances they are prescribed as low vision aids, especially following cataract surgery, when results are less than expected and patients need optical boosters for their defective sight. Many of these patients find regular glasses too distorting, hazardous, or unsuitable in their work. For them, their contact lenses are classified as *prosthetic* devices, and as such, their cost may be reimbursed by Medicare.

Refinements in contact lens designs have come swiftly since the Food and Drug Administration approved them for marketing in the 1970s—soft contact lenses, lenses that could be left in the eyes for weeks, bifocal contacts, new products for lens cleaning and care. Optical experts predict that improvements in contact lens design and in precision manufacturing processes will reduce the incidence of eye irritation and facilitate easier lens care.

Before the 1950s children born with severe eye defects were shunted into schools for the blind or sequestered at home. Today, pediatric surgery saves thousands of children from blindness. Cataracts are removed, vitrectomy clears debris that impedes sight, and "natural lenses" are grafted on corneas of infants born without lenses or whose congenital cataracts have been removed. Too young for plastic lens implants, or for managing eyeglasses, these infants receive "living contact lenses" surgically, donor corneal tissue sewed to the infant's own cornea.

Though pediatric eye surgery is preventing blindness, seldom does surgery enable the child's eyes to function perfectly. Nor is corrective surgery available to the majority of visually impaired infants and young children. The lucky few who benefit from these operations are overbalanced by the increasing number of children whose lives are saved by "heroic measures," but who are doomed to marginal lives in which incurable sight loss is only one of many defects. As this segment of the population grows, it has become an increasing concern to dedicated child-care professionals.

Dr. Anne L. Corn, assistant professor in education of the visually handicapped, University of Texas, at Austin, says there is a lack of qualified teachers to "habilitate" these children in residential schools or in their own homes. Even those children who, despite several handicaps, are able to attend regular schools need attention from specially trained professionals qualified to evaluate functional vision and train the children in getting about and coping with classroom situations. According to Dr. Corn, future prospects for the increasing number of multihandicapped children with visual impairments are dim unless the education establishment recognizes the special needs of this segment of our society and promotes recruitment and training of teachers and counselors.

Prospects for visually impaired adults are brighter. They are attracting the attention of national, state and local agencies formerly committed to serving only the blind. An example of the shift of emphasis from the totally blind to the partially sighted is in the Minnesota State Services for the Blind, one of the first state agencies in the country to develop a staff training program for low vision services.

This program, developed with the guidance of the Pennsylvania College of Optometry, stems from a survey of counselors on the staff of the Minnesota State Services for the Blind. Respondents to the survey identified low vision rehabilitation service training as the number-one priority. The enthusiastically backed, carefully planned training course is expected to be a model for other state agencies for the blind that are moving into providing rehabilitation services for the partially sighted.

Simulation technology, commonly used by the aerospace industry and the military to train aircraft pilots and astronauts, is being applied to visualizing what partially sighted patients actually see. According to Dr. Gregory L. Goodrich, research psychologist at the Veterans Administration Medical Center in Palo Alto, California, where some of this research has been carried out, the great value of this technology in the field of low vision is that it makes possible the production of films or videotapes that show graphically what the partially sighted person sees. "That is," says Dr. Goodrich, "the technology can accurately simulate functional vision. This has enormous implications for the training of rehabilitation professionals. Beyond that, this technique can help families and the general public understand the effects various disorders have on vision."

Dr. Goodrich also sees future applications of vision simulation technology in improving the low vision specialist's ability to assess functionally an individual's visual capacity. More than that, this technology will help vision education specialists develop training methods that will help the partially sighted use their vision to best advantage. Another spin-off will be its contribution to the improved design of low vision aids.

As a researcher himself, Dr. Goodrich values vision-simulation technology as a research tool, enabling vision investigators, using computer images, to control the visual environment in studies and make possible the replication of findings. "In this way," says Dr. Goodrich, "the current status of low vision research as a 'soft science' can be transformed into 'hard science,' which will make the field more attractive to a wider range of clinical and basic researchers, whose work will have an impact on developments in low vision services."

Dr. Gerald R. Friedman, director of low vision services at Retina Foundation, says that the next decade will produce many more different types of aids that will be more than magnifiers. He predicts microprocessors designed for more than reading printed or typed materials. Far more sophisticated aids are now on the drawing boards. As the partially sighted become more proficient in using computers, they will rely on them more extensively to gain access to information and program them to talk to one another, opening up whole areas of communication that bypass visual restrictions.

Not only will low vision services expand, Dr. Friedman predicts, but clinics will pay more attention to cost-effectiveness. Studies of cost-effectiveness, while contributing to more efficient management, can be used to show the financial advantages of public funding for services to the visually impaired, especially to the elderly whose visual impairments prevent their functioning independently.

With funds from the federal Administration on Aging, the New York Lighthouse, which had been serving the blind for seventy-nine years, conducted a pilot project on vision and aging in five localities across the country. Titled "A Better View of You," the project, a partnership between eye-care clinicians and human-services professionals, aimed at encouraging the elderly to be their own advocates for vision care. As a result of this pilot project, the New York Lighthouse in 1985 set up the National Center for Vision and Aging to promote the rehabilitation of the visually impaired.

Directed by Arlene Gordon, associate executive director of the Lighthouse, the Center, besides coordinating services, research and training, is a clearinghouse for information on vision care for the elderly, not only collecting information, but disseminating it through community education programs and professional training. Blazing a trail in vision education is the Center's program of working with corporations. Members of the Center's staff work with corporate personnel in the medical, human resources, preretirement and employee-assistance departments, providing them with educational materials, training and information about community low vision clinics and other resources.

Private and public agencies for the blind will be with us for some time, but in recent years they have been shifting their emphasis from blindness to sightedness as the number of totally blind declines and agencies acknowledge the needs of millions of partially sighted Americans. The American Foundation for the Blind, possibly the largest agency for the blind in the world, has taken the leadership in supporting services for the partially sighted.

In 1985, the Foundation published a pamphlet entitled *Low Vision Questions and Answers: Definitions, Aids, Services,* a document that significantly draws the distinction between blindness and low vision. Answering the question "Are persons with low vision blind?" the pamphlet states: "The American Foundation for the Blind suggests that the term 'Blind' and 'Blindness' be reserved for persons who have no usable sight at all, and the terms 'visually impaired' or 'low vision' be used for persons who have some usable vision, no matter how little."

That is a distinction low vision specialists have been making all along, but for the Foundation to put it into print had great importance for the low vision movement. The Foundation has on its staff a low vision consultant who publicizes the low vision concept through articles and public appearances. In 1985, the Foundation appointed a low vision task force, headed by Dr. Randall T. Jose, to develop a definition of low vision as a basis for setting standards for low vision services and for justifying third-party payments—Medicare and other reimbursements for low vision services and visual aids.

Looking to the future, administrators, educators, clinicians, consultants from colleges of optometry and ophthalmology, and vision researchers identify these needs as low vision moves into a new phase.

- A national association of low vision professionals.
- Centralized sources (national, regional and local) for information about low vision services.
- Guidelines for setting up and managing low vision clinics and centers.
- A redefinition of "legal blindness" (originally termed "occupational blindness").
- A definition of blindness in relation to low vision.
- Statistics on number of partially sighted in the United States.
- Public education about the nature and values of low vision services, types of clinics and centers, and how to find them.
- Criteria for eligibility of partially sighted for rehabilitation services. (The partially sighted complain about being railroaded into programs designed primarily for the totally blind.)
- Closer ties between businesses and low vision service providers. (The New York Lighthouse corporate liaison program is a prototype for this kind of activity.)
- Liaison between optical-aid industry and low vision clinicians.
- Education program for legislators on economic value of low vision services and need for "third party payments."
- Stepped-up recruitment and training of professionals in all low vision activities.

Even as this book was being written, the demand for low vision services exceeded resources. But every day, in low vision clinics, eye-care departments of medical centers, and offices of private practitioners in low vision, men and women, boys and girls, small children and infants are being kept out of the blindness system through new ways of assessing usable vision, the prescription of appropriate aids, and intelligent referrals for surgical or other medical correction of visual defects.

Meeting the escalating demands for low vision services will require a major coordinated effort—eye-care professionals, optical and nonoptical aid providers, eye researchers, rehabilitation trainers, and educators, all working together to help the millions of Americans with low vision use the sight they have with optimum efficiency.

APPENDIX

References and Resources

From the hundreds of references I used in writing this book, I have selected a few I think will be especially interesting and helpful.

BOOKS

Brown, Barbara B. *New Mind, New Body: Bio-Feedback: New Directions for the Mind.* New York: Harper & Row, 1975.

Carroll, Thomas J. *Blindness: What It Is, What It Does, and How to Live with It.* Boston: Little, Brown, 1961.

Chevigny, Hector. *My Eyes Have a Cold Nose.* New Haven, CT: Yale University Press, 1946.

Cholden, Louis S. *A Psychiatrist Works with Blindness.* New York: The American Foundation for the Blind, 1958.

DiStasi, Lawrence. *Mal Occhio (Evil Eye): The Underside of Vision.* San Francisco: North Point Press, 1981.

Faye, Eleanor E. *Clinical Low Vision.* Revised edition. Boston: Little, Brown, 1984.

Fonda, Gerald E. *Management of Low Vision.* New York: Thieme-Stratton, 1981.

Goffman, Erving. *Stigma.* Englewood Cliffs, NJ: Prentice-Hall, Inc., 1963.

Henri, Robert. *The Art Spirit.* New York: J. B. Lippincott, 1930.

Huxley, Aldous. *The Art of Seeing.* New York: Harper & Brothers, 1942.

Jose, Randall T., ed. *Understanding Low Vision.* New York: The American Foundation for the Blind, 1983.

MacCurdy, Edward, ed. *The Notebooks of Leonardo da Vinci.* New York, George Braziller, 1954.

Mehta, Ved. *Vedi.* New York: Oxford University Press, 1982.

Potok, Andrew. *Ordinary Daylight.* New York: Holt, Rinehart & Winston, 1980.

Powis, David. *The Signs of Crime: A Field Manual for Police.* Maidenhead, Berkshire, England: McGraw-Hill Book Co. (UK), 1977.

Scott, Robert A. *The Making of Blind Men.* New Brunswick, NJ: Transaction, 1981.

Shulman, Julius. *Cataracts: The Complete Guide—from Diagnosis to Recovery—for Patients and Families.* New York: Simon and Schuster, 1984.

Trevor-Roper, Patrick. *The World Through Blunted Sight: An Inquiry into the Influence of Defective Vision on Art and Character.* Indianapolis and New York: Bobbs-Merrill, 1970.

Weisse, Fran A., and Mimi Winer. *Coping with Sight Loss: The Vision Resource Book.* Watertown, MA: Vision Foundation, 1986.

CATALOGS—AIDS AND PRODUCTS FOR THE VISUALLY IMPAIRED

American Printing House for the Blind
1839 Frankfort Avenue
Louisville, KY 40206

Independent Living Aids, Inc.
11 Commercial Court
Plainview, NY 11803

IRTI—Innovative Rehabilitation Technology, Inc.
26699 Snell Lane
Los Altos Hills, CA 94022

Large Type Books in Print
R. R. Bowker
P.O. Box 1807
Ann Arbor, MI 48106

LS&S Group
P.O. Box 673
Northbrook, IL 60065

PRODUCTS FOR PEOPLE WITH VISION PROBLEMS

American Foundation for the Blind
15 West 16th Street
New York, NY 10011

Reading Materials in Large Type (Ref. Circular, June 1983)
National Library Service for the Blind and Physically Handicapped
The Library of Congress
Washington, DC 20542

Vis/Aids, Inc.
86-30 102nd Street
Richmond Hill, NY 11418

Vision Aids Resource Guide
Science Products
Box A
Southeastern, PA 19399

Vision Insight Products
Bossert Specialties Co.
P.O. Box 15441
Phoenix, AZ 85060

Vision Resource List—1986 Edition
Vision Foundation, Inc.
818 Mt. Auburn Street
Watertown, MA 02172

Visual Aids and Informational Material
National Association for Visually Handicapped
305 East 24th Street
New York, NY 10010

CATALOGS—RECORDED BOOKS

Audio Cassette Catalog
Ingram Audio
347 Reedwood Drive
Nashville, TN 37217

Books on Tape
Box 71405
Atlantic Richfield Station
Los Angeles, CA 90071

Guide to Spoken-Word Recordings: General Nonfiction
National Library Service for the Blind and Physically Handicapped
The Library of Congress
Washington, DC 20542

Mind's Eye
Great Books on Cassettes
4 Commercial Boulevard
Novato, CA 94947

Recorded Books
6306 Aaron Lane
Clinton, MD 20735

SBI Publishers in Sound, Inc.
48 Willow Street
South Lee, MA 02160

Talking Books Topics
Bi-monthly listing of books added to the Library of Congress national talking book collection
National Library Service for the Blind and Physically Handicapped
Library of Congress
Washington, DC 20542

Note: Book stores and libraries have copies of recorded books and catalogs.

COMPUTER SYSTEMS APPROPRIATE FOR THE VISUALLY IMPAIRED

Note: The computer systems listed here are those most frequently mentioned by partially sighted users. The ferment in the computer industry—companies going out of business, mergers, new developments in computer technology—guarantees constant changes in any list. Computer companies are offering special attachments and capabilities that adapt standard computers for use by the visually impaired. The advice given by low vision specialists in computer use is first, decide what you want the computer to do for you, then shop around for the type of computer and the software program that suits your purposes. Don't be misled by people (salesmen included) who tell you you can learn to use the computer effectively in fifteen minutes. You will need instruction.

You may obtain information about their computer products by writing to these companies:

Apollo Lasers, Inc.
20932 Lassen Street
Chatsworth, CA 91311

Computer Aids Corp.
Technology for the Print Handicapped
4929 South Lafayette Street
Fort Wayne, IN 46806

Kurzweil Computer Products, Inc.
185 Albany Street
Cambridge, MA 02139

Sensory Aids Corp.
205 West Grand Avenue
Bensenville, IL 60106

Telesensory Systems, Inc.
Low Vision Products
455 North Bernardo Avenue
P.O. Box 7455
Mountain View, CA 94039

Vtek, Inc.
1625 Olympic Boulevard
Santa Monica, CA 90404

COMPUTER TRAINING CENTERS FOR THE VISUALLY IMPAIRED

Computer Center
Carroll Center for the Blind
770 Centre Street
Newton, MA 02158

C-TEC Center
Sensory Aids Foundation
399 Sherman Avenue
Palo Alto, CA 94306

STORER Computer Access Center
Sight Center
Cleveland Society for the Blind
1909 East 101 Street
Cleveland, OH 44106

DIRECTORIES

Directory of Agencies Serving the Visually Handicapped in the U.S. (Current Edition) American Foundation for the Blind, 15 West 16th Street, New York, NY 10011

Library Resources for the Blind and Physically Handicapped (Current Edition) National Library Service for the Blind and Physically Handicapped, The Library of Congress, Washington, DC 20542

GUIDELINES FOR ORGANIZING SUPPORT GROUPS

Guidelines for Organizing Self-Help Groups, by Mimi Winer.
Vision Foundation
818 Mt. Auburn Street
Watertown, MA 02172

A Roadmap to Organizing C.C.L.V. Chapter/Support Groups, by Sarita Williams.
Council of Citizens with Low Vision
337 South Sherman Drive
Indianapolis, IN 46201

Self-Help Center: A National Resource
1600 Dodge Avenue—Suite S-122
Evanston, IL 60201

LOW VISION CLINICS—HOW TO FIND ONE

The primary source of information about low vision clinics should be your eye doctor, but at the rate low vision clinics are being established, ophthalmologists and optometrists do not always have up-to-date information about them. You may have to do some searching yourself. A logical place to start is the phone book. Some phone books list the clinics under a general heading "Vision." Not all clinics are designated "clinics." Some are listed as low vision centers, vision rehabilitation centers, low vision services. Some are in departments of ophthalmology in medical schools, others in colleges of optometry. Now that public and private agencies for the blind are branching out into services for the partially sighted, those agencies are a likely source of information about low vision clinics. Other sources of information about the clinics are state commissions for the blind, local rehabilitation agencies, ophthalmology departments in hospitals and medical schools, and local and county medical societies.

MANUALS, PAMPHLETS AND FACT SHEETS

Aids for the 80s: What They Are and What They Do, by C. Michael Mellor, American Foundation for the Blind (AFB), 15 West 16th Street, New York, NY 10011

Answers to Frequently Asked Questions about Low Vision, by Paul B. Freeman and Barbara J. Freeman, The Center for Vision Rehabilitation, 1500 Brodhead Road, Aliquippa, PA 15001

Dealing with the Threat of Loss, by Dorothy H. Stiefel, Booklet No. 1, The Business of Living Booklets, P.O. Box 8388, Corpus Christi, TX 78412

Eye Trumpets: A Consumer Guide to Low Vision and Low Vision Aids, by Bill Carroll. Low Vision Association of Ontario, 145 Adelaide Street West, Toronto, Ontario M5H 3H4, Canada

The First Steps: How to Help People Who Are Losing Their Sight, by the staff of Peninsula Center for the Blind, Palo Alto, CA 94303

Know Your Eyes, Fact Sheet. National Eye Institute, National Institutes of Health, Bethesda, MD 20892

Low Vision, Illustrated pamphlet prepared by the Low Vision Clinic of the School of Optometry, University of Alabama in Birmingham, University Station, Birmingham, AL 35294

Low Vision, Fact Sheet. National Eye Institute, National Institutes of Health, Bethesda, MD 20892

Low Vision Questions and Answers: Definitions, Aids, Services, American Foundation for the Blind, 15 West 16th Street, New York, NY 10011

Making Life More Livable: Simple Adaptations for the Homes of Blind and Visually Impaired Older People, by Irving R. Dickman. American Foundation for the Blind, 15 West 16th Street, New York, NY 10011

Optometric Low Vision Care News Backgrounder, Communications Division in cooperation with the Low Vision Section of the American Optometric Association, 243 North Lindbergh Blvd., St. Louis, MO 63141

Voice Indexing: Procedure for Sequential Voice Indexing on a 2-Track or 4-Track Cassette Recorder. For visually impaired, rehabilitation counselors and teachers, and special education teachers in schools, homes and clinics. Voice Indexing for the Blind, Inc., 9116 St. Andrews Place, College Park, MD 20740

Note: Voice indexing has practical applications also for the sighted—students, writers, reporters who use tape recorders.

What Can We Do about Limited Vision? by Irving R. Dickman. Public Affairs Pamphlet #491. Public Affairs Pamphlets, 381 Park Avenue South, New York, NY 10016

Large Print Book Club
The Doubleday Large Print Home Library
Garden City, NY 11535-1104

ORGANIZATIONS—SOURCES OF INFORMATION ABOUT IMPAIRED VISION

American Academy of Ophthalmology
1822 Fillmore Street
P. O. Box 7424
San Francisco, CA 94120

American Council of the Blind
1010 Vermont Avenue-Suite 1100
Washington, DC 20005

American Foundation for the Blind
15 West 16th Street
New York, NY 10011

American Optometric Association
243 North Lindbergh Boulevard
St. Louis, MO 63141

Association for Education and Rehabilitation of the Blind and Visually Impaired
206 North Washington Street—Suite 320
Alexandria, VA 22314

Committee on Vision
National Research Council
2101 Constitution Avenue
Washington, DC 20418

Eye Institute of the Pennsylvania College of Optometry
13th & Spencer Streets
Philadelphia, PA 19141

Eye Research Institute of Retina Foundation
20 Staniford Street
Boston, MA 02114

International Association of Lions Clubs
300 22nd Street
Oak Brook, IL 60521

National Association for Visually Handicapped
305 East 24th Street, Suite 17-C
New York, NY 10010

National Council of Citizens with Low Vision
337 South Sherman Drive
Indianapolis, IN 46201

National Library Service for the Blind and Physically Handicapped
Library of Congress
Washington, DC 20542

National Society for the Prevention of Blindness
79 Madison Avenue
New York, NY 10016

New York Lighthouse Low Vision Service
111 East 59th Street
New York, NY 10022

Partially Sighted Society
Southern and Western Regional Association for the Blind
55 Eton Avenue
London NW3 3ET
England

Rehabilitation Services Administration
Division for Blind and Visually Impaired
330 C Street
Washington, DC 20201

RP Foundation
8331 Mindale Circle
Baltimore, MD 21207

Texas Association of Retinitis Pigmentosa
P.O. Box 8388
Corpus Christi, TX 78412

Veterans Administration
Services for Blind and Visually Impaired Veterans
810 Vermont Avenue
Washington, DC 20420

Vision Foundation, Inc.
818 Mt. Auburn Street
Watertown, MA 02172

PERIODICALS

AFB News
American Foundation for the Blind
15 West 16th Street
New York, NY 10011

The Braille Forum
American Council of the Blind
1010 Vermont Avenue, Suite 1100
Washington, DC 20005

C.C.L.V. News
Council of Citizens with Low Vision
337 South Sherman Drive
Indianapolis, IN 46201

Dialogue: The Magazine for the Visually Impaired
Quarterly
Large type, disc and braille
Dialogue Publications, Inc.
3100 Oak Park Avenue
Berwin, IL 60402

Journal of Vision Rehabilitation
University of Houston
College of Optometry
4800 Calhoun
Houston, TX 77004

Magazines in Special Media: Subscription Sources
Reference Circular, January 1985
National Library Service for the Blind and Physically Handicapped
The Library of Congress
Washington, DC 20542

Sundial
Eye Research Institute of Retina Foundation
P.O. Box 9041
20 Staniford Street
Boston, MA 02114

TARP
Texas Association of Retinitis Pigmentosa
P. O. Box 8388
Corpus Christi, TX 78412

REPORTS

Annual Reports. Research to Prevent Blindness, 1982, 1983 and current. Research to Prevent Blindness, 598 Madison Avenue, New York, NY 10022

Cataract Surgery: Fraud, Waste, and Abuse. A Report. Subcommittee on Health and Long-term Care of the Select Committee on Aging, House of Representatives, 99th Congress, July 19, 1985. Committee Publication No. 99-506. U.S. Government Printing Office, Washington, DC 20402

Light for Low Vision. Proceedings of the Symposium cosponsored by the Chartered Institution of Building Services, Lighting Division, and by the Partially Sighted Society, April 4, 1978. Partially Sighted Society, Southern and Western Regional Association for the Blind, 55 Eton Avenue, London NW3 3ET, England.

OSHA Oversight—Video Terminals in the Workplace. Hearings before the Subcommittee on Health and Safety of the Committee on Education and Labor, House of Representatives, 98th Congress. February 28; March 13; April 3; May 1, 8, 15; June 5 and 12, 1984. U.S. Government Printing Office, Washington, DC 20402

The Use of Residual Vision by Visually Disabled Persons. Report on World Health Organization's international meeting on partial sight, Brussels, January 28–30, 1981. EURP Reports and Studies No. 41. World Health Organization, Distribution and Sales Service, 1211 Geneva, Switzerland.

INDEX